THE *Ultimate*
HIGH PROTEIN
HANDBOOK

C000245145

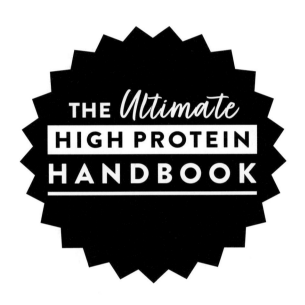

THE *Ultimate*
HIGH PROTEIN
HANDBOOK

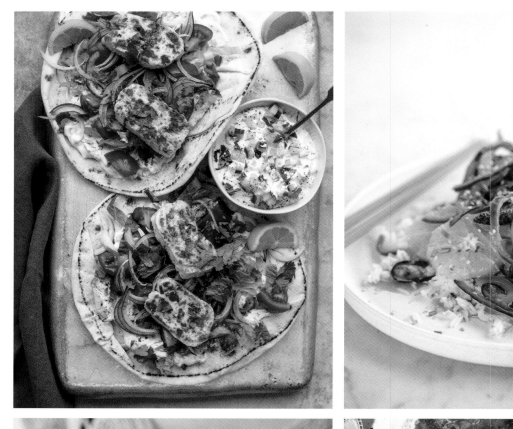
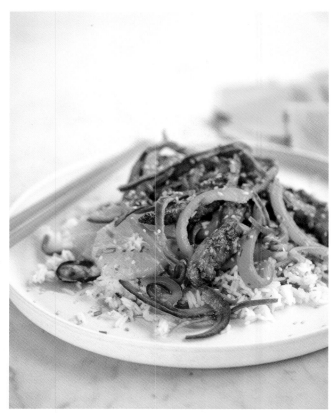
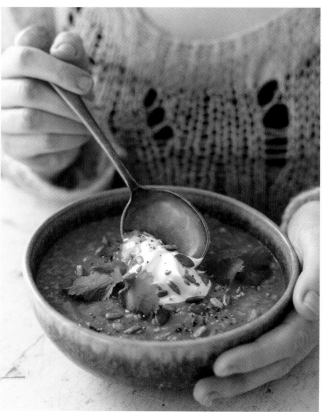
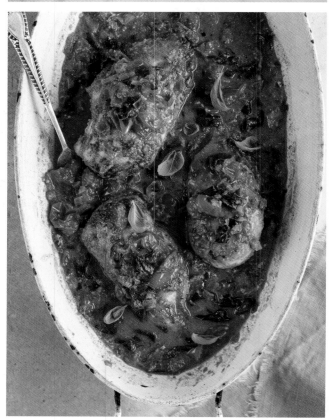

SCOTT BAPTIE

THE *Ultimate* HIGH PROTEIN HANDBOOK

80 HEALTHY, DELICIOUS, EASY RECIPES FOR ALL THE FAMILY

Harper
North

CONTENTS

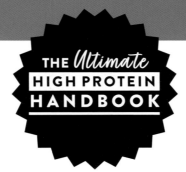

INTRODUCTION

My name is Scott. If we've never met or spoken before, I'll keep this intro quick and say I'm a nutritionist, weight loss coach and recipe creator. My aim is to make healthy eating as easy as possible for you, which means cutting through the nutrition nonsense, forgoing the fads and showing you how to eat well without listening to the 'noise' about all the foods you should either supposedly avoid or fear.

The Ultimate High Protein Handbook is for people who want to enjoy easy, high-protein, family-friendly recipes without spending hours slaving in the kitchen or hunting down obscure ingredients you can't find in the supermarket. I've seen so many healthy cookbooks that get the green tick from me when I'm wearing my nutritionist hat but sadly get a big red cross when it comes to practicality, flavour and all-round pleasure. Nobody really has the time to cook two meals an evening: a 'healthy' meal for yourself and then something else that the kids or your other half will actually eat because otherwise the healthy option is kale, kale and more kale. Wouldn't it just be much easier if the 'healthy meal' was actually one that everyone wanted to eat? In our household we serve one meal at dinner time. It's always nutritious – protein-packed and flavoursome – it doesn't take hours to prepare, and my wife and our three-year-old love it! We all eat the same thing: the only thing that needs to be changed is the portion size (more about that later).

But why high-protein, I hear you ask? Even if you're not trying to be the next Arnold Schwarzenegger, eating more protein is an easy and tasty way to level up your diet. One of the key benefits to eating more protein is that it can help to regulate your appetite and keep those hunger pangs at bay. This is because 1) protein-rich foods generally take more time to break down in your stomach compared to carbohydrates and fat and 2) when you eat protein, your ghrelin levels (a hormone that makes you feel hungry) drops and another hormone, peptide YY (a hormone that helps you to feel full and satisfied), increases. Therefore, if you're trying to lose weight through eating fewer calories than normal, by simply eating more protein you can help control your appetite and stay feeling fuller for longer. Studies have shown that increasing protein intake by 15 per cent can help people eat fewer calories overall without even specifically trying to eat less.

Eating more protein is also great if you want to help your body to recover faster after exercise, reduce age-related muscle loss, improve bone health and get stronger. It's probably the closest thing to a 'superfood' that exists. And the best thing? You don't have to pay over the odds for it, nor hunt down an uber-specific health food shop. You can load your trolley with protein at your local supermarket and this book will show you 80 delicious ways how to cook it without spending hours in the kitchen.

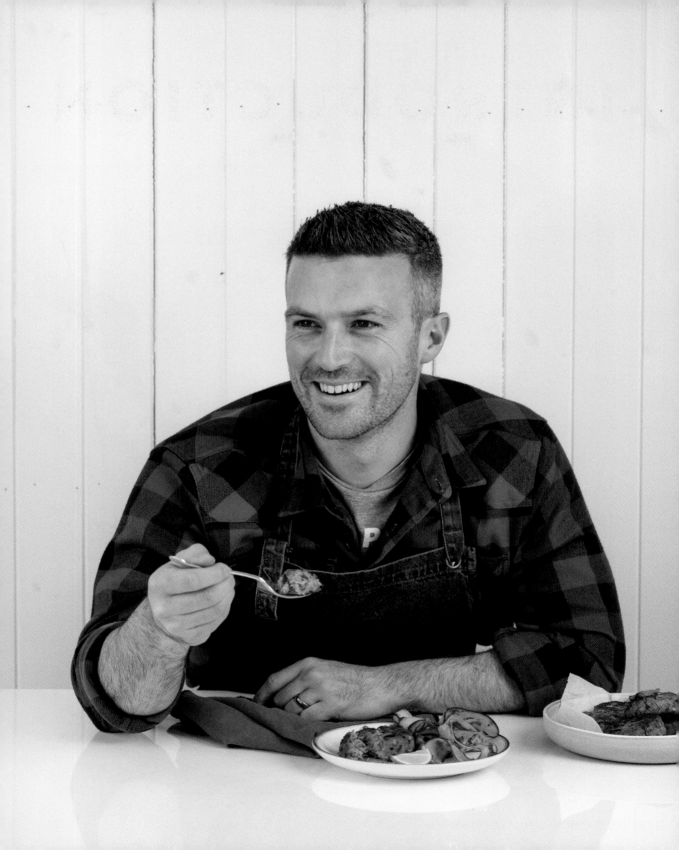

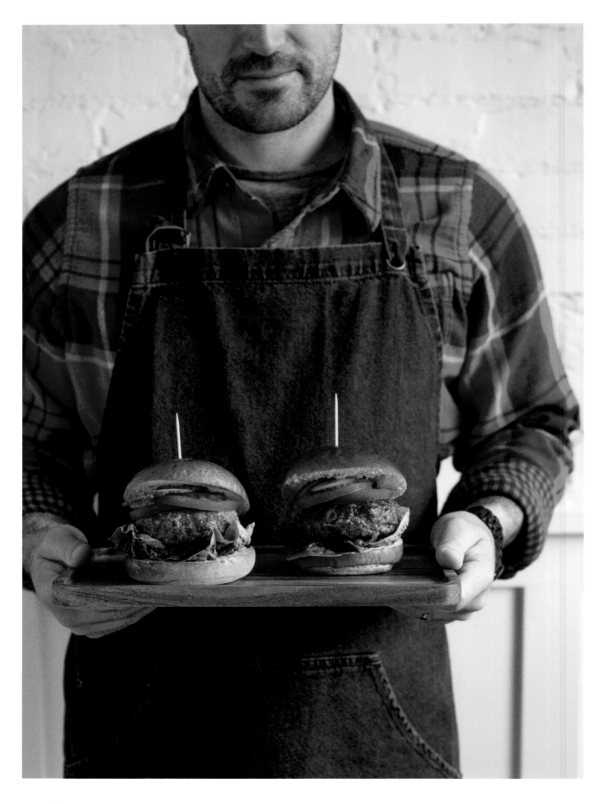

KEEP IT SUPER SIMPLE

The problem with recipe books, especially the ones that purport to be 'healthy', is that in many cases you end up spending vast amounts of time trawling expensive speciality food shops or forking out cash online for random ingredients that you only ever use once. Himalayan moss extract anyone? If you're like me, you probably like doing all your shopping in one supermarket, and quite cheaply at that. So I've done my best to make sure that you'll be able to find every ingredient you need in this recipe book in your weekly shop.

If you're trying to eat more healthily, convenience and ease is key to long-term success. So I've tried to pack this book with stuff that's easy to find, prepare and cook, without breaking the bank. What's more, each recipe has all the nutrition information included. If you use an app to track your calories or macros, you'll find a helpful barcode for each recipe to scan the meal straight into your food diary. Winner winner, high-protein dinner.

In my view, keeping your dishes to a single core element is crucial to making things easy is rather than making elaborate sauces, sides and garnishes. So what you'll find here are single-dish recipes, organised by meal type rather than by ingredient, occasion, lunar phase or any other unnecessary device.

We kick things off with breakfasts and brunches, then there are lighter meals, main meals (sorted by main ingredient) and some tasty snacks at the end.

You can easily have some of the breakfasts or brunches for a main meal, of course. Do what you fancy and remember that flexibility is key. Speaking of which, most of the recipes are designed so that the main ingredient can be swapped out – pork for chicken, for instance – as long as you remember to adjust the cooking time accordingly. You might also choose to cook some things in an air fryer instead of the oven, or you could make a casserole in the slow cooker. All of this is generally fine as long as you make sure everything is cooked through.

But if you do make changes to the recipe it will have an impact on the calories, macronutrients etc. Leaving out some garlic or adding an onion isn't going to make much of a difference. But using chicken thighs (which are much fattier and higher in calories) instead of chicken breasts, will have a more significant impact. For some that'll be fine; for anyone counting calories it's something to pay attention to.

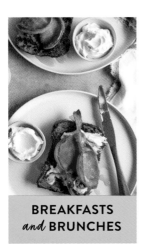

BREAKFASTS and BRUNCHES

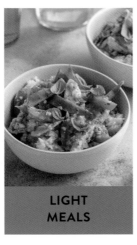

LIGHT MEALS

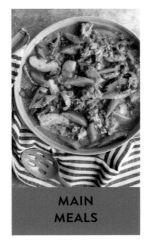

MAIN MEALS

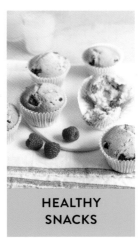

HEALTHY SNACKS

THE SKINNY ON SIDE DISHES

You'll see that some of the dishes in this book are a 'complete' meal with some kind of meat, maybe a sauce, vegetables and carbohydrates all included. Others will just feature the main component. Again, the aim is to give you plenty of flexibility when putting your meals together. We all require a different number of calories to keep us going and to support whatever goal it is we are working towards. I figured that if I just gave you a complete meal every time, it wouldn't offer as much wiggle room to customise. Some folks will want a lower carb diet, others might be on fewer calories, whereas some people will be trying to add muscle or may have very large calorie requirements and need to slam the carbs with every meal.

Therefore, most of the time, what you decide to serve with the meal is entirely up to you. In order to make most square meals as balanced as possible this will probably mean a decent whack of protein (provided by the recipes here), some veg (if the recipe doesn't have a lot included already) and some kind of carbohydrate on the side. Carbs are not evil, neither are they inherently 'unhealthy'. As always, it comes down to portion control and understanding that when I am referring to a side of carbs it most likely means rice, pasta, couscous, potato etc, and not jelly babies. Cool?

SCALING MEALS UP OR DOWN

The meals in the book generally do provide around four portions, with some serving less, and some serving more. So you might be wondering about scaling meals up or down depending on how many portions, or mouths you need to feed? For most things it's just a case of doubling or halving but for spicy meals, specifically when it comes to using chilli powder or flakes, you should take care. Dried chilli doesn't scale well and if you just double up you might find the meal much hotter than expected. If scaling anything up that's spicy, err on the side of caution and just go for what's in the recipe, plus a tad more unless you want to spend the evening panting and dabbing your forehead.

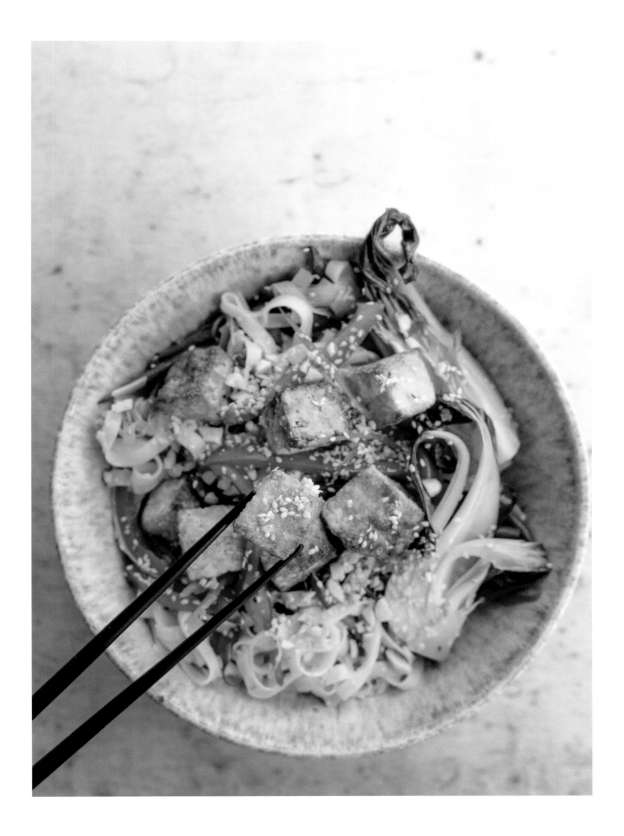

THINGS TO MAKE COOKING EASIER

In the interests of keeping things simple, here are three items and ingredients that will make life a bit easier when it comes to most recipes in this book.

1. DIGITAL SCALES.

These are much better than old-school analogue ones, especially for measuring lower weights. If you don't have some, you can pick up a trusty set pretty cheaply.

2. AIR FRYER.

Until you actually own an air fryer, you probably won't be entirely sure what one is. Basically we're talking a very small oven that heats up in a matter of minutes, reduces cooking times by about 30 per cent and makes anything that's meant to be crispy, super crispy – almost like it's been deep fried. We use ours several times per week for things like goujons, breads, potato wedges, etc. Don't worry, there are only two or three recipes in this book that use an air fryer, and I provide alternative cooking methods if you don't have one. But trust me, you won't regret buying one.

3. GARLIC AND GINGER PASTE.

If I include garlic and ginger in the same recipe, they're usually in equal amounts. The reason for this is simply convenience. I try to avoid peeling garlic and ginger as it takes up half the prep time. Instead, I have a big tub of garlic and ginger paste – that's one tub, not two separate ones – in the fridge. It keeps for absolutely ages. These tubs are staples in any Indian takeaway restaurant and you can find them quite easily online, but you can also get smaller jars in the supermarket. Get some and thank me later.

GRAMS, TABLESPOONS AND DIGITAL SCALES

I'm always in a quandary about whether I should list some of the ingredients as tablespoons/teaspoons, etc or just give specific weights. Here I have generally favoured the spoons approach (so you won't need to get the scales out all the time) if it's a small volume of liquid or something very light (like spices). But I've gone for scale weight for other ingredients such as garlic, etc. Hopefully you'll agree this is a happy medium. If in doubt, an ingredient measured using a teaspoon (tsp) usually weighs around 5g and a tablespoon (tbsp) usually weighs around 12-15g.

BARCODES

You'll see barcodes at the foot of the page for each recipe. These are included so you can quickly and easy scan in the nutritional information to your chosen calorie counting app, either Nutracheck or MyFitnessPal.

DON'T SWEAT THE SMALL STUFF

Cooking should be fun. Healthy eating should improve the quality of your life, not detract from living an enjoyable one. So don't sweat the small stuff, ok? This is particularly relevant for people who are tracking calories or counting their macros. What I mean by this is, don't worry if your measurements are a bit off when you're cooking. If the recipe says to use 150g of chicken and you use 170g, who cares? If you use a bigger onion than usual, it doesn't matter. Seriously, don't miss the forest for the trees. Remember that even when the calories are listed on a food label there is a +/- 15% degree of error. And this is fine. You don't need to be that specific with your measurements so just relax.

Some people have asked me how heavy a cooked portion of one of my recipes should be. Firstly, the cooked weight of a recipe is going to vary tremendously depending on how much water was lost when you cooked it, the ingredients you used, etc. Secondly, this is extreme micromanagement. When it comes to divvying up the portions, just eyeball it. You don't need to get the scales out to make sure each portion is exactly 437.5g. Yes, some of your portions will be bigger, some smaller so your calories (if tracking) might not be exactly as you planned, but given what I said about the high margin of error on food labels anyway it's not a big deal. Combine this with the fact that studies have repeatedly shown we generally underestimate the calories we consume anyway it's really not going to make or break your fitness progress if your portions aren't exact.

Happy Cooking, and Good Luck — Scott

PART 1
BREAKFASTS

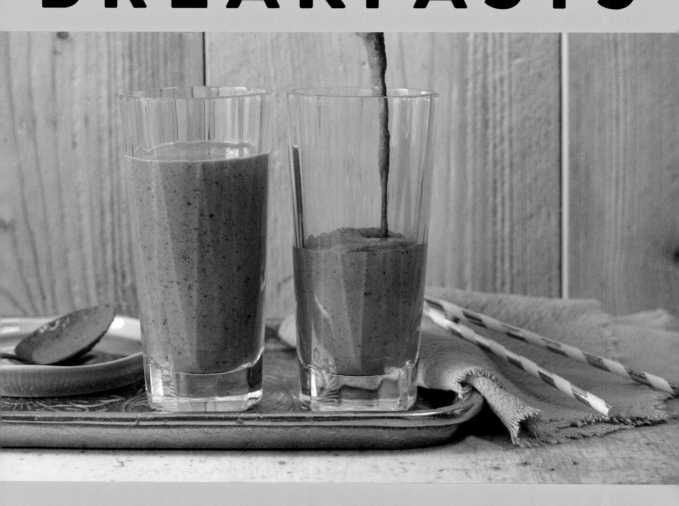

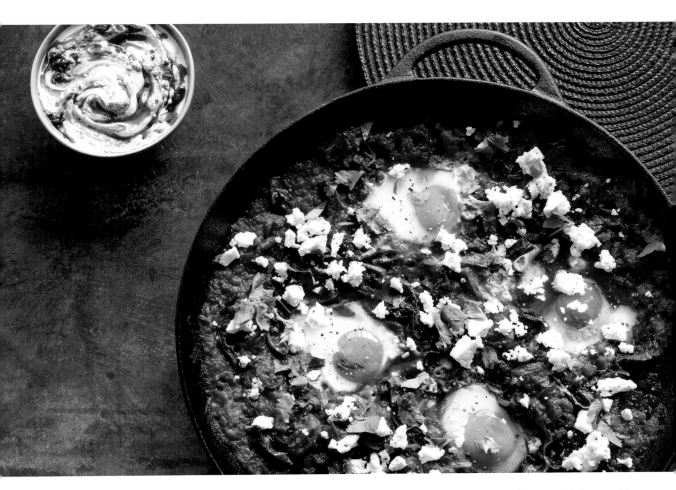

and BRUNCHES

THE *Ultimate*
HIGH PROTEIN
HANDBOOK

IF YOU'RE FED UP OF SCRAMBLED EGGS FOR A 'HEALTHY BREAKFAST' LOOK NO FUTHER. THERE'S A SELECTION OF DELICIOUS HIGH-PROTEIN BREAKFASTS FOR YOU TO TRY THAT AREN'T JUST EGGS COOKED EVERY WAY UNDER THE SUN! YES, EGGS DO FEATURE HEAVILY IN THIS SECTION – IT'S HARD NOT TO INCLUDE THEM AS THEY'RE SUCH A GREAT SOURCE OF PROTEIN. BUT HOPEFULLY YOU'LL BE ABLE TO USE THEM IN SOME RECIPES YOU'VE NEVER HAD BEFORE RATHER THAN JUST SCRAMBLING, BOILING AND POACHING THEM.

I'VE ALSO INCLUDED THE EXACT BREAKFAST I HAVE ABOUT 360 DAYS OF THE YEAR (BORING, I KNOW). NOW YOU MAY HAVE HEARD THAT 'BREAKFAST IS THE MOST IMPORTANT MEAL OF THE DAY', THIS ISN'T REALLY TRUE BUT THE SCIENCE DOES SHOW US THAT PEOPLE WHO DO EAT BREAKFAST, SPECIFICALLY PROTEIN AT BREAKFAST, HAVE BETTER APPETITE CONTROL AND EATING HABITS AS THEY GO THROUGHOUT THE DAY.

BREAKFAST SMOOTHIE

466
CALORIES
per serving

I am a creature of habit and over the past ten years I've probably started my day with this breakfast 99 per cent of the time. It's a great choice if you work out in the morning. It's generally easier to digest food if it's partially broken down (as in a smoothie), so when exercising in the morning I find this gives you a good hit of protein and carbs without sitting on your stomach and feeling uncomfortable. If you take any supplements in powder form (greens, creatine, etc), then they can easily be added to this. At the weekend I go wild and add a tablespoon of peanut butter.

INGREDIENTS

50g porridge oats
70g frozen berries (any)
1 scoop of protein powder (around 25g)
250ml semi-skimmed milk

Simple one this . . . add to blender and blitz.

**Nutritional info
per serving:**
Calories: 466kcal
Protein: 38g
Carbs: 56g
Fat: 10g

Prep time: 2 minutes
Serves: 1

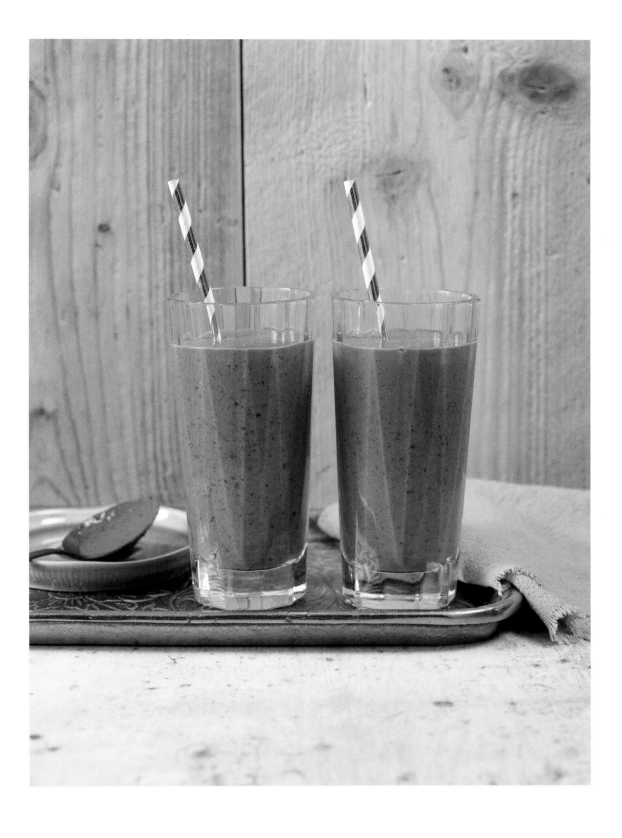

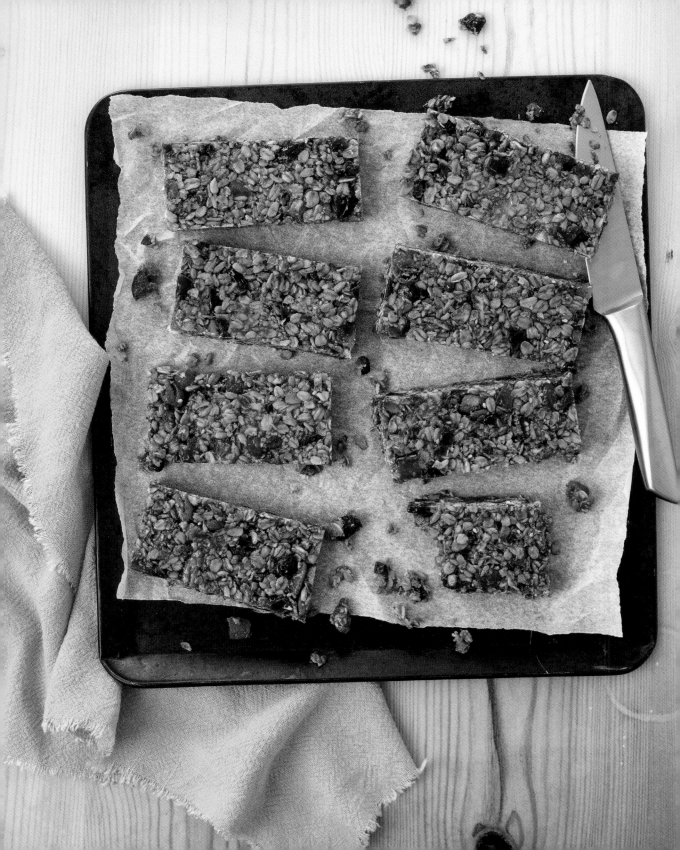

CRUNCHY BREAKFAST BARS

400
CALORIES
per bar

These delicious fruit and nut bars are great for breakfast on the go. I sometimes nibble one if I need a protein boost later in the day. To increase the protein content, add some protein powder to the mixture before baking.

INGREDIENTS

300g porridge oats
150g chopped pecans or walnuts
100g ready-to-eat dried apricots, chopped
100g stoned dates, ideally mejdool dates, chopped
60g dried cherries or cranberries
4 tbsp mixed seeds, eg pumpkin, sunflower, sesame, chia
60g dark chocolate chips
150g butter, plus extra for greasing
7 tbsp clear honey
Few drops of vanilla essence

Preheat the oven to 160°C (140°C fan)/315°F/gas 3. Lightly butter a shallow 30 x 20cm baking tin and line with greaseproof paper.

Put the oats, nuts, dried fruits, seeds and chocolate in a large mixing bowl and stir to mix well and distribute everything evenly.

Put the butter and honey in a small pan and set over a low heat. Stir gently with a wooden spoon until the butter melts and combines with the honey.

Pour over the oat mixture and add the vanilla essence, then mix well. If the mixture is too sticky and not firm enough, just stir in some more oats until you get the right consistency. If it's too dry, stir in some more melted butter or nut butter.

Spoon the mixture into the lined baking tin and smooth the top with a palette knife or by pressing down with the back of a spoon. Bake for 25–30 minutes, or until crisp and golden brown on top.

Remove from the oven and allow to cool slightly in the tin before cutting into 12 bars. Leave in the tin until completely cold, then transfer the bars to a sealed tin or airtight container. Eat within 5 days.

Nutritional info per bar:

Calories: 400kcal
Protein: 7g
Carbs: 39g
Fat: 24g

Prep time: 20 minutes
Cook time: 25–30 minutes
Makes: 12 bars

1 169920 245058

HOMEMADE CRUNCHY GRANOLA BOWLS

612 CALORIES per serving

Homemade granola is healthier than most shop-bought varieties as it has less sugar. Adding nut butter (peanut, almond, cashew or hazelnut) boosts the protein content. This recipe makes enough for eight servings, but you could make double the amount and keep the granola in an airtight container, as it will stay crisp for up to three weeks.

INGREDIENTS

5 tbsp smooth nut butter
2 tbsp coconut oil
4 tbsp maple syrup
1 tsp ground cinnamon
350g porridge oats
75g chopped almonds
60g mixed seeds, eg pumpkin and sunflower seeds
4 tbsp chia seeds
100g raisins

Topping

8 tbsp Greek yoghurt or dairy-free coconut yoghurt
8 tbsp coconut flakes
400g blackberries or chopped apricots

Preheat the oven to 170°C (150°C fan)/325°F/gas 3. Line a baking tray with greaseproof paper.

Put the nut butter, coconut oil, maple syrup and cinnamon in a saucepan and set over a low heat. Stir gently for 2–3 minutes or until melted and smooth.

Add the oats, nuts and seeds and stir until everything is coated. If it's too dry, just add some maple syrup. Pour the mixture on to the lined baking tray and spread it out evenly.

Bake in the oven for 25–30 minutes, turning halfway through, until golden brown. Remove from the oven and set aside. Don't worry if the granola isn't very crisp – it will get crisper and crunchy as it cools. When cold, stir in the raisins and transfer to a sealed container.

Serve the granola in bowls topped with yoghurt, coconut flakes and fresh fruit.

Nutritional info per serving:
Calories: 612kcal
Protein: 17g
Carbs: 64g
Fat: 32g

Prep time: 10 minutes
Cook time: 25–30 minutes
Makes: approx. 500g granola (8 servings)

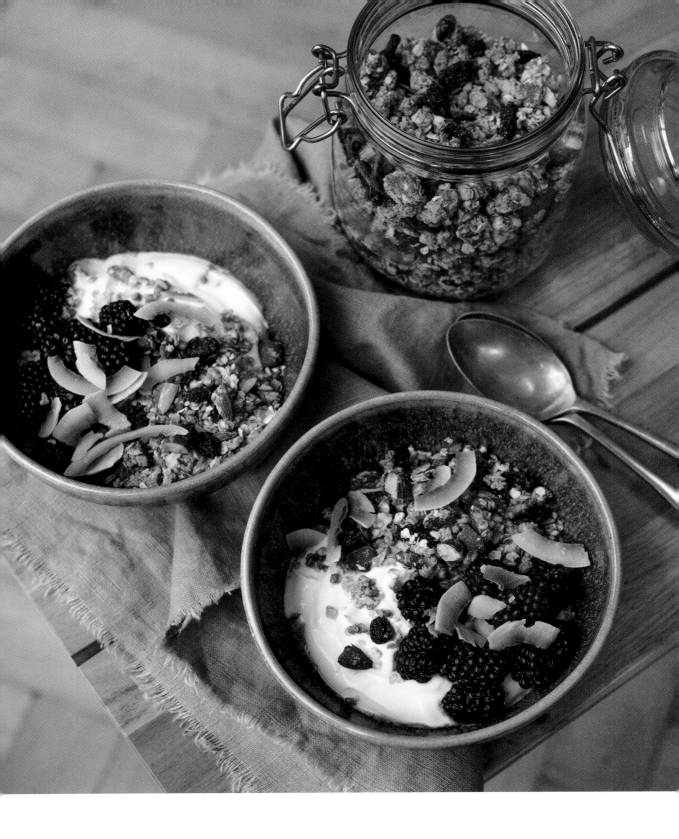

OVERNIGHT OAT *and* YOGHURT CHIA POTS

473
CALORIES
per serving

These nutritious breakfast pots are so quick and easy to make. Just mix everything up before you go to bed and chill in the fridge overnight. By the following morning, the oats and chia seeds will have swelled up in the milk and yoghurt to create a wonderfully creamy dish to start the day. Serve with nuts and berries or a topping of your choice.

I know chia seeds are a bit of a stereotypical 'health food' but they have an amazing ability to absorb approximately ten times their dry weight, so when you add them to a liquid they swell and thicken it to a porridge-like consistency. They are a powerhouse of nutrients and an excellent source of protein.

INGREDIENTS

250g 0%-fat Greek yoghurt
500ml milk (use any dairy or plant-based milk, eg nut, oat or soya)
1 tbsp agave or maple syrup
180g porridge oats
4 tbsp chia seeds
Grated zest of 1 sweet juicy orange

Topping

200g raspberries
4 tbsp chopped nuts, eg walnuts, hazelnuts or almonds
4 tbsp 0%-fat yoghurt

Put the Greek yoghurt, milk, syrup, porridge oats, chia seeds and orange zest in a bowl. Stir well until everything is thoroughly mixed.

Divide the mixture between four wide-mouthed glass Mason jars or clear glass or plastic containers. Cover with the lids or some cling film and chill in the fridge overnight.

The following morning, uncover the jars and top with the raspberries, chopped nuts and a spoonful of yoghurt.

Nutritional info per serving:
Calories: 473kcal
Protein: 26g
Carbs: 54g
Fat: 17g

Prep time: 10 minutes + overnight to chill
Serves: 4

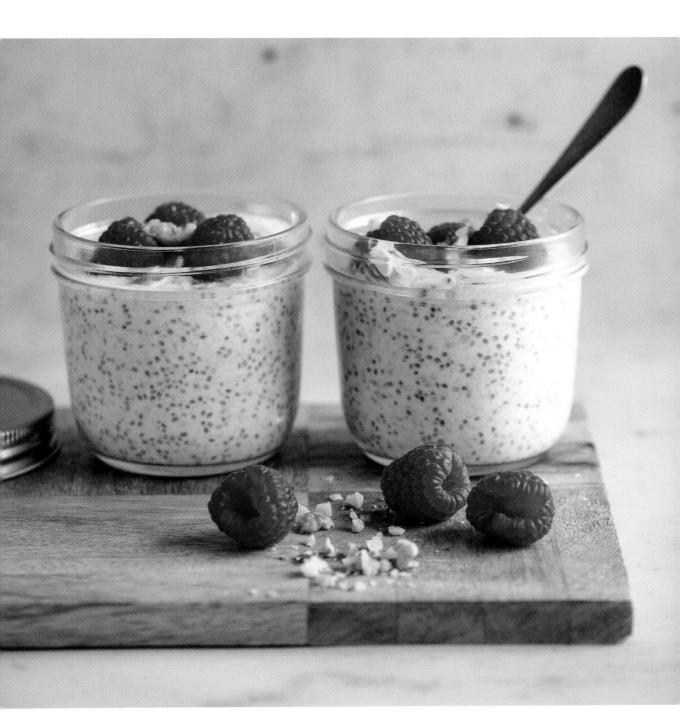

SAVOURY BREAKFAST MUFFINS

193
CALORIES
per muffin

Bake a batch of these delicious veggie muffins for a quick breakfast when you're in a hurry or want a healthy snack. They're the perfect way to add more vegetables to your diet. For the best and lightest results, don't over-mix the muffin mixture. Be gentle and fold in the cheese, vegetables, seeds and nuts.

INGREDIENTS

2 tbsp olive oil, plus extra for greasing
1 red onion, grated or finely chopped
150g spinach leaves, washed, trimmed and chopped
Few sprigs of fresh flat-leaf parsley, chopped
250g wholemeal self-raising flour
1 tsp bicarbonate of soda
Pinch of sea salt
2 medium free-range eggs
250g 0%-fat Greek yoghurt
115g grated low-fat cheddar cheese, plus extra for sprinkling
2 large carrots, grated
3 tbsp mixed seeds, eg poppy, sunflower, pumpkin, chia
3 tbsp pine nuts

Preheat the oven to 200°C (180°C fan)/400°F/gas 6. Line a 12-hole muffin pan with paper cases.

Heat the oil in a saucepan set over a medium heat and cook the onion, stirring occasionally, for 6–8 minutes, or until softened. Add the spinach and cook for 1–2 minutes until the leaves wilt. Stir in the parsley and remove the pan from the heat.

Sift the flour, bicarbonate of soda and salt into a large bowl. Beat the eggs and yoghurt together and stir into the flour. Add the cooled onion and spinach mixture, then gently fold in the cheddar, carrot, seeds and pine nuts.

Spoon the mixture into the paper cases and sprinkle with grated cheese. Bake for 18–20 minutes, or until the muffins are risen and golden brown. They are cooked when a thin skewer inserted into the centre comes out clean.

Leave to cool on a wire rack. The muffins are best eaten lukewarm or at room temperature. They will stay fresh stored in a sealed container for 2–3 days.

Nutritional info per muffin:
Calories: 193kcal
Protein: 12g
Carbs: 16g
Fat: 9g

Prep time: 20 minutes
Cook time: 30 minutes
Makes: 12 muffins

7 870926 988422

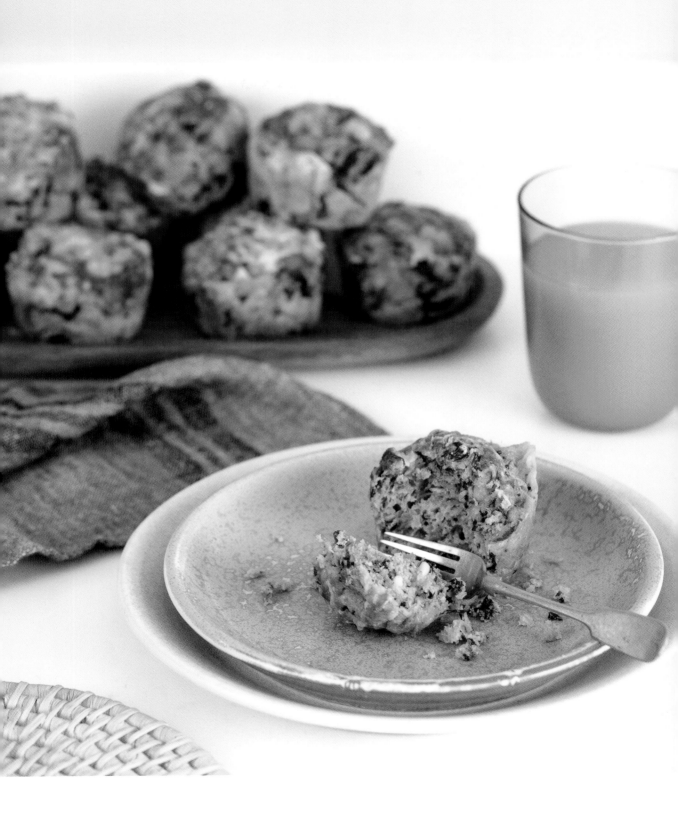

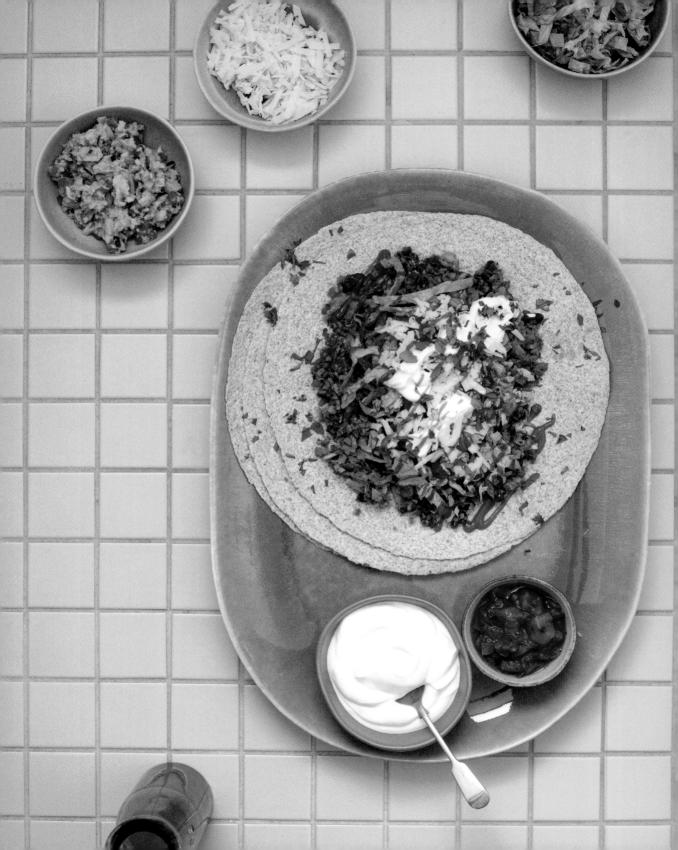

BREAKFAST BURRITOS

If you like spicy food, these Mexican burritos are the perfect breakfast. They're simple to make and ideal for eating 'on the go'. Or you can take one with you for a packed lunch – they're so versatile. If you don't have tinned refried beans in the cupboard, no problem. Just mash some tinned kidney beans, black beans or even white cannellini or butter beans. If you don't have time to make the smashed avocado, substitute with shop-bought, ready-made guacamole. Oh, and if you happen to have any leftover roast chicken from the weekend, that's also a great addition.

INGREDIENTS

1 tbsp olive oil
Bunch of spring onions, sliced
1 hot red chilli, diced
400g tin refried beans
3–4 tbsp cold water
Handful of fresh coriander, chopped
4 large wholewheat tortillas or wraps
1 small cos lettuce, trimmed and shredded
4 tbsp hot spicy tomato salsa
4 heaped tbsp Greek yoghurt
100g grated low-fat cheddar cheese
Hot sauce, for drizzling (optional)
Salt and pepper

Smashed avocado

1 medium ripe avocado, peeled and stoned
1 small red onion, finely chopped
3 tinned chipotle peppers in adobo sauce, diced
Juice of ½ lime
Sea salt crystals

Heat the olive oil in a non-stick frying pan set over low to medium heat. Cook the spring onion and chilli, stirring occasionally, for 6 minutes, or until tender. Add the refried beans and cold water. Cook gently for 5 minutes, stirring occasionally, and then stir in the coriander. Season to taste with salt and pepper.

While the bean filling is cooking, make the smashed avocado: use a fork to mash the avocado in a bowl – not too smooth as you want it to have some texture. Stir in the red onion, chipotle peppers and lime juice. Season to taste with sea salt.

Warm the tortillas on a lightly oiled griddle pan or frying pan set over low heat. Watch them carefully so they don't get crispy or catchy.

Spread the shredded lettuce over the warm tortillas, not right up to the edge. Cover with the smashed avocado, tomato salsa, yoghurt, grated cheese and hot sauce, if using.

Roll up the tortillas or fold the ends over the filling to enclose it and then roll. Serve immediately or store in a sealed container in the fridge for a few hours.

Nutritional info per serving:
Calories: 475kcal
Protein: 19g
Carbs: 66g
Fat: 15g

Prep time: 15 minutes
Cook time: 12 minutes
Serves: 4

6 743733 202825

SHAKSHUKA

541
CALORIES
per serving

This traditional dish of eggs poached in a spicy tomato sauce is often served for breakfast throughout the Middle East and North Africa. It's also perfect for a light lunch or dinner. Don't be put off by the long list of ingredients – you'll have most of them in your kitchen cupboards or fridge. If you don't like coriander, use flat-leaf parsley instead. You can also swirl some pomegranate molasses, harissa or sweet chilli sauce into the yoghurt.

INGREDIENTS

2 tbsp olive oil
1 red onion, diced
2 red peppers, chopped
3 garlic cloves, crushed
1 red chilli, shredded
1 tsp smoked paprika
1 tsp ground cumin
2 x 400g tins chopped tomatoes
2 tbsp tomato purée
Pinch of sugar
100g spinach leaves, washed, trimmed and shredded
Handful of fresh coriander, chopped
4 large free-range eggs
150g low-fat feta cheese
Salt and pepper

To serve

250g low-fat Greek yoghurt
1 tbsp hot sauce, eg Sriracha
4 warm wholewheat pitas or flatbreads

Heat the oil in a large frying pan set over a medium heat. Add the onion, red pepper, garlic and chilli and cook, stirring occasionally, for 5 minutes, or until tender. Stir in the ground spices and cook for 1 minute.

Add the tomatoes, tomato purée and sugar and simmer for 10–15 minutes, or until the sauce starts to reduce and thicken. Season to taste with salt and pepper and stir in the spinach and half of the coriander.

With the back of a spoon, make four hollows in the sauce and break an egg into each one. Cover the pan and simmer gently for 8–10 minutes, or until the eggs are cooked – the whites should be set and the yolks still slightly runny. Crumble the feta over the top and sprinkle with the remaining coriander.

Divide between four shallow serving bowls and serve immediately with a bowl of yoghurt swirled with hot sauce on the side, and some warm pita or flatbreads to soak up the spicy tomato sauce.

**Nutritional info
per serving:**
Calories: 541kcal
Protein: 33g
Carbs: 46g
Fat: 25g

Prep time: 15 minutes
Cook time: 25–30 minutes
Serves: 4

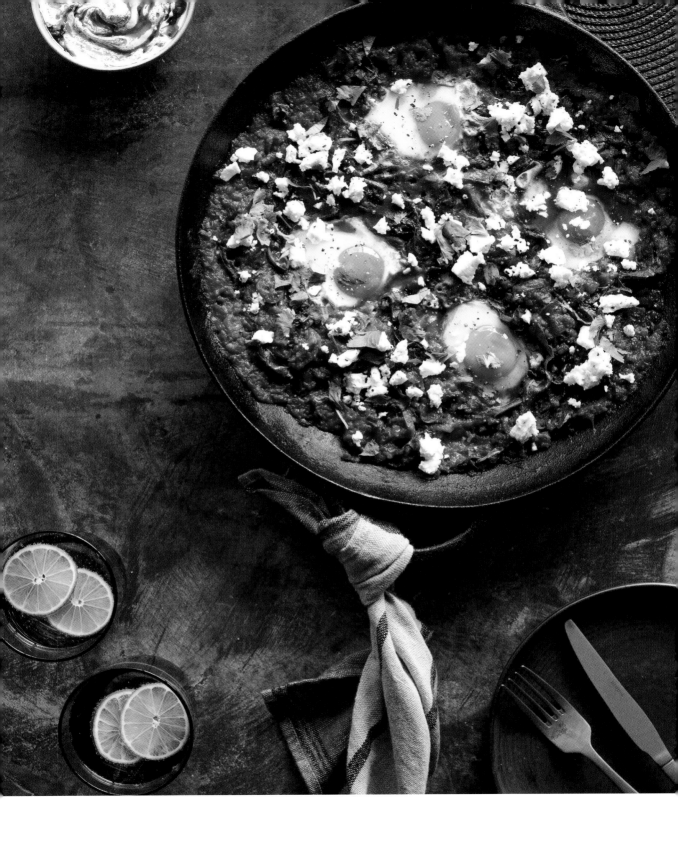

CILBIR

This is inspired by the Turkish breakfast dish of poached eggs and served with dill-flavoured yoghurt and fiery harissa. It's surprisingly quick and easy to prepare and packed with protein and nutrients to get your day off to a good start. If you're hungry, serve two poached eggs per person and you'll have even more protein per serving. Don't crack the eggs directly into the pan in case they break – you want them to stay whole. Alternatively, you can use an egg poacher if you're the kind of person who has an egg poacher. You could also use kale instead of spinach, or even frozen spinach. If you like even more heat, add a few chilli flakes or smoked paprika to the melted butter.

INGREDIENTS

400g spinach leaves, washed and trimmed
1 tbsp water
1 tbsp white wine vinegar
4 medium free-range eggs
500g low-fat Greek yoghurt
3 garlic cloves, crushed
2 tsp harissa paste
60g butter, melted
Few sprigs of fresh dill, finely chopped
4 large wholewheat pita breads, warmed

Put the spinach in a large saucepan with the water. Cover with a lid and set over a medium heat. Cook for 2–3 minutes, giving the pan an occasional shake, until the leaves wilt and turn bright green. Drain in a colander and return to the pan to keep warm.

Set a wide saucepan of water over a high heat and bring to the boil. Add the vinegar and reduce the heat to a simmer. Gently crack an egg into a bowl, then slide it carefully into the simmering water. Repeat with the three remaining eggs. Poach each egg for 3–4 minutes until the whites are set and the yolks are still runny. Remove carefully with a slotted spoon and drain on kitchen paper.

Heat the yoghurt and garlic in a small pan set over the lowest possible heat, so the yoghurt doesn't separate.

Place the spinach in four serving bowls and spoon the yoghurt over the top. Swirl in a little harissa. Top with a poached egg and pour over the melted butter. Sprinkle with dill and serve immediately with warm pita breads to wipe up the spicy yoghurt and egg yolk.

Nutritional info per serving:
Calories: 457kcal
Protein: 31g
Carbs: 36g
Fat: 21g

Prep time: 5 minutes
Cook time: 10 minutes
Serves: 4

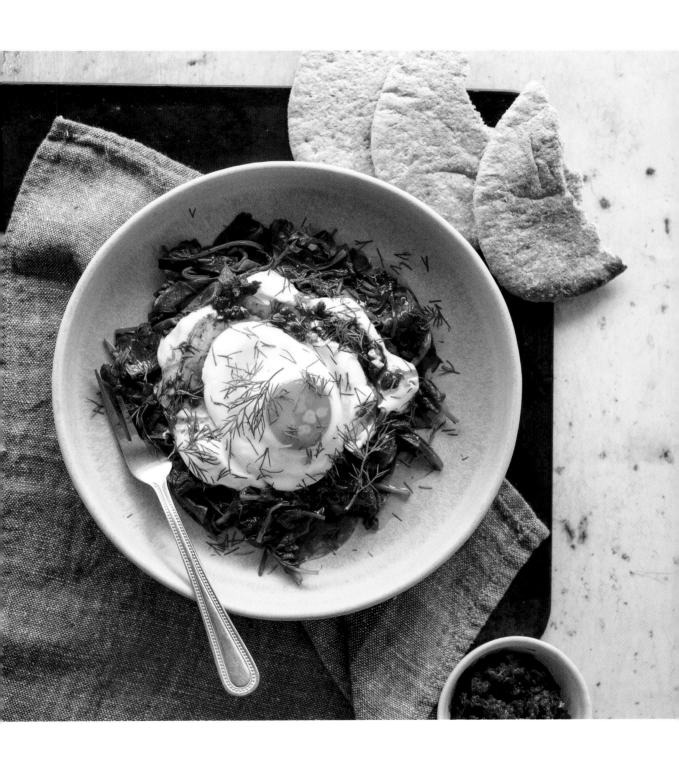

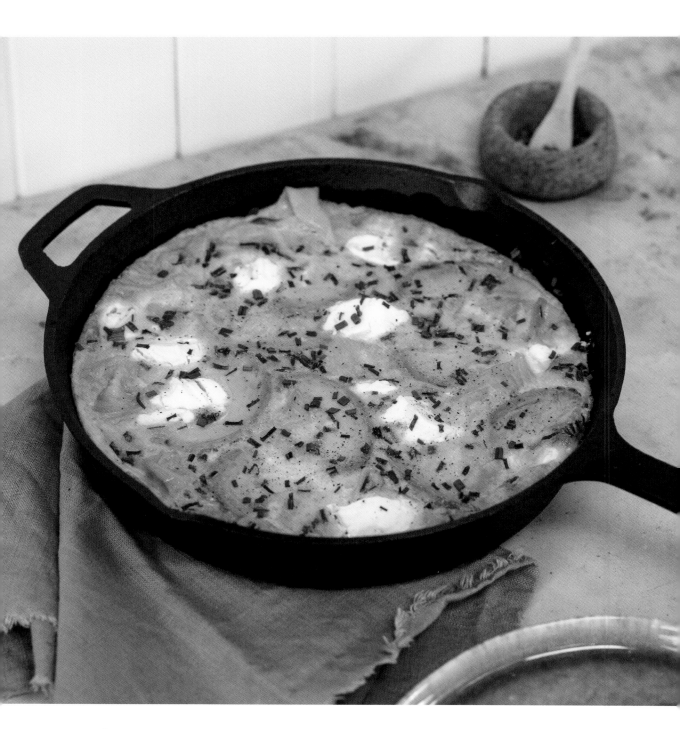

SMOKED SALMON
and CHIVE OMELETTE

Nutrient-dense eggs and salmon are always a tasty combo. As well as being rich in protein, the salmon is a good source of essential omega-3 fatty acids, which are good for heart, brain and joint health. This is more of a frittata than a classic omelette, as it's easier and less tiring to cook everything in one pan rather than stand over the hob making individual omelettes! Don't buy expensive smoked salmon – most supermarkets sell cheaper smoked salmon trimmings, which are equally tasty and nutritious. They are ideal for making omelettes or adding to scrambled eggs. If you don't like salmon, you've probably not read this far … but if you don't like smoked salmon, add some diced ham or crumbled crispy bacon instead.

INGREDIENTS

8 medium free-range eggs
2 tbsp milk
Small bunch of fresh chives, snipped
30g unsalted butter
1 medium ripe avocado, peeled, stoned and
  diced
200g smoked salmon, chopped
100g low-fat soft cheese
Salt and pepper

Beat the eggs with the milk and a little salt and pepper in a large bowl. Stir in the chives.

Melt the butter in a large frying pan set over a low heat. When it starts to sizzle, pour in the beaten eggs and swirl them around the pan, tilting it to cover the base. As the omelette starts to set underneath, draw it in towards the centre with a wooden spoon, so the liquid egg runs out over the pan to the edges.

Cook for 3–4 minutes until the omelette is starting to turn golden underneath and then gently stir the avocado, smoked salmon and teaspoonfuls of the soft cheese into the runny egg. Cook for 1–2 minutes, or until starting to set on top and golden-brown underneath.

Pop the omelette under a preheated hot grill to brown and set the top. Watch it carefully – it only needs 1–2 minutes maximum. Alternatively, just fold the omelette over the filling, cook for 1 minute and then slide it out of the pan.

Cut the omelette into four portions and serve immediately.

Nutritional info per serving:
Calories: 407kcal
Protein: 29g
Carbs: 3g
Fat: 31g

Prep time: 10 minutes
Cook time: 10 minutes
Serves: 4

1 281011 206592

WHOLEGRAIN FRENCH TOAST *and* CRISPY BACON

492 CALORIES per serving

French toast is so easy to make and perfect for weekend brunches. Even people who aren't keen on eggs seem to love this. I usually serve it drizzled with maple syrup but a crunchy peanut butter drizzle (see below) packs an extra protein punch.

INGREDIENTS

3 medium free-range eggs
5 tbsp milk (use any dairy or plant-based milk, eg nut, oat or soya)
Few drops of vanilla extract
½ tsp ground cinnamon
4 thick slices wholegrain or multiseed bread
Unsalted butter, for frying
8 rashers back bacon
2 tbsp maple syrup
115g low-fat soft cheese
Salt and pepper

Beat the eggs, milk, vanilla and cinnamon together in a shallow bowl. Season with salt and pepper.

Dip the slices of bread (both sides) into the egg mixture and leave just long enough for the egg mixture to penetrate the bread (usually less than 1 minute or 30 seconds each side). Don't leave them for too long or the bread will become soggy and fall apart.

Heat the butter in a large non-stick frying pan set over a low to medium heat. When it's really hot, carefully add 2 slices of soaked bread and cook for 2–3 minutes until crisp and golden brown underneath. Turn the slices over and cook the other side. Remove and keep warm while you fry the remaining slices in the same way.

Meanwhile, cook the bacon in another frying pan over a medium to high heat until browned and crispy.

Serve the French toast drizzled with maple syrup, with the crispy bacon and soft cheese. Alternatively, use the peanut butter drizzle below.

Put the maple syrup and peanut butter in a small pan and stir gently over a low heat until melted and well combined. Drizzle over the French toast.

Nutritional info per serving (with PB drizzle):
Calories: 492kcal
Protein: 26g
Carbs: 34g
Fat: 28g

Prep time: 6–8 minutes
Cook time: 8–12 minutes
Serves: 4

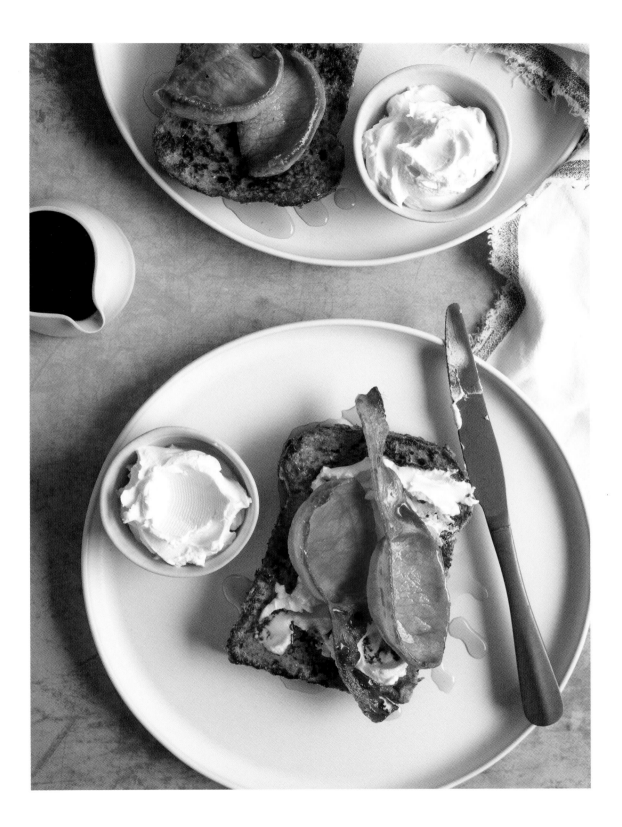

PART 2
LIGHT

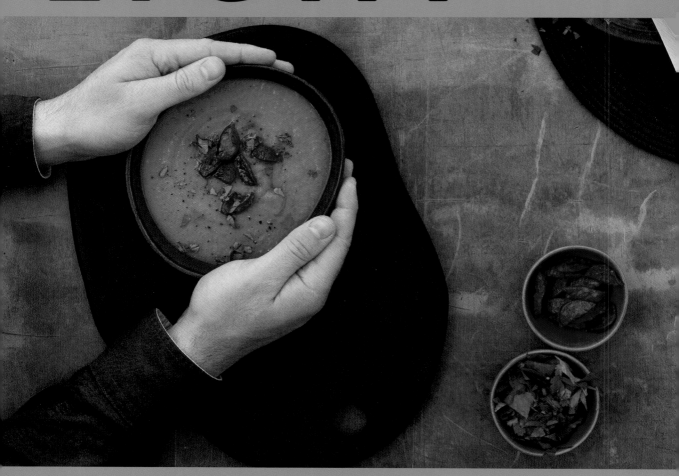

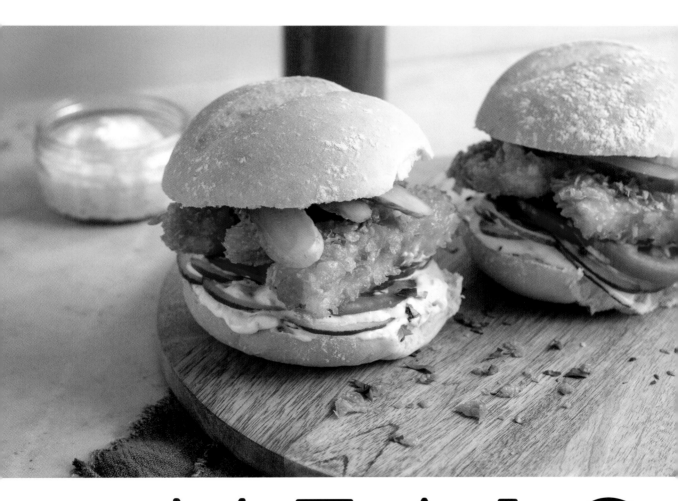

MEALS

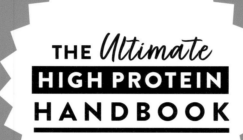

IN THIS SECTION I'VE INCLUDED SOME OF THE MEALS THAT WOULD WORK WELL AS LUNCHES, WOULD TASTE GREAT EATEN OUTSIDE ON A SUMMERS EVENING OR JUST FOR WHEN YOU WANT SOMETHING THAT'S LIGHT, FRESH AND EXTREMELY TASTY. WE'VE GOT SALADS, SOUPS, WRAPS, KEBABS, SANDWICHES AND MORE.

MOST OF THE RECIPES ARE BRAND NEW BUT MY FOLLOWERS WILL RECOGNISE A FEW OF THE MOST POPULAR RECIPES LIKE MY FAVOURITE SOUP OF ALL TIME – SWEET POTATO AND CHORIZO – FOUND ON PAGE 60. IF YOU'VE NOT MADE IT BEFORE, IT'S A GREAT PLACE TO START. THE SPICY SALMON BURGERS WERE ONE OF MY WIFE'S FAVOURITE RECIPES IN THE BOOK AND MY BROTHER LOVED THE LIGHTER TUSCAN CHICKEN TOO. THERE'S LOTS FOR YOU TO GET STUCK IN TO.

30-MINUTE CHICKEN
and BACON RISOTTO

436
CALORIES
per serving

I can't always find the time and energy to make a risotto – mine's a more of the throw-it-in-the-pan-and-leave-it approach to cooking. But add chicken and bacon to it and my oven version of a risotto becomes pretty irresistible. Because this recipe uses the oven instead of cooking it on the hob, I suppose it's probably more of a biryani or pilaf, but we're all more familiar with risotto as a concept hence the name.

INGREDIENTS

1 tbsp olive oil
6 rashers bacon (fat removed), chopped
4 chicken breasts, chopped
1 red onion, chopped
1 green pepper, chopped
200g risotto rice
750ml chicken stock
100g cherry tomatoes, halved

Heat the oven to 180°C (160°C fan)/350°F/gas 4.

Place a large ovenproof pan on the hob over a medium to high heat and add the olive oil, bacon, chicken breasts, onion and pepper.

Cook for several minutes until the chicken starts to brown.

Add the uncooked rice to the pan, stir and continue to fry for a further minute.

Add the stock and tomatoes to the pan, cover and cook in the oven for around 30 minutes or until all the stock has been absorbed and the rice has cooked. If you need to add a splash more water or stock to the pan during cooking to make sure the rice is cooked fully, then please do so.

**Nutritional info
per serving:**
Calories: 436kcal
Protein: 43g
Carbs: 48g
Fat: 8g

Prep time: 5 minutes
Cook time: 40 minutes
Serves: 4

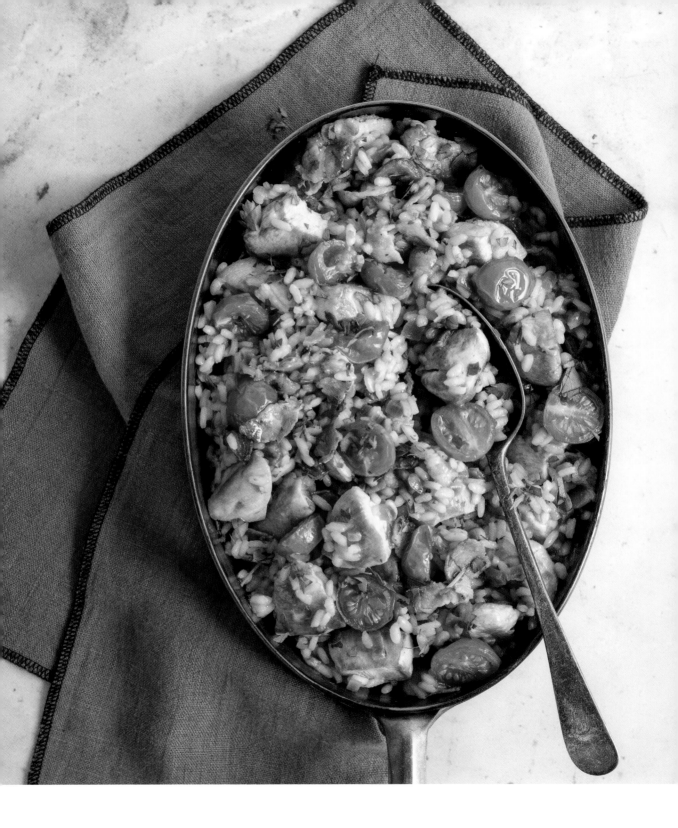

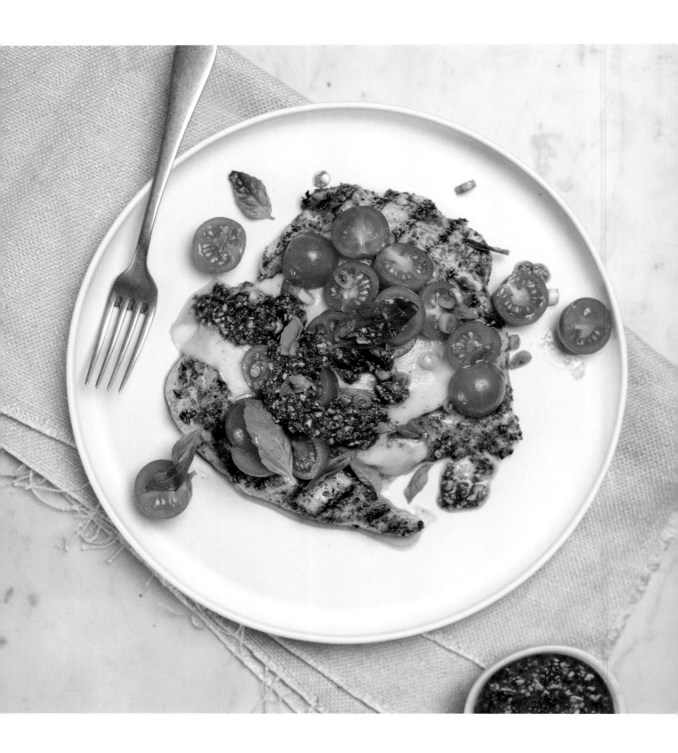

BASIL *and* MOZZARELLA CHICKEN

This is a great summer dish. I love the tomato and basil salad on its own, let alone with the mozzarella chicken. As always when cooking a recipe that involves marinating, the longer you leave it, the better. I've written 30 minutes into the method, but if you can leave it overnight, or at least for a couple of hours, you're going to get an even more flavoursome dish.

INGREDIENTS

Chicken
½ tsp garlic powder
½ tsp mixed herbs
½ tsp onion powder
1 tbsp olive oil
1 tsp balsamic vinegar
Few grinds of black pepper
500g chicken breasts, bashed into steaks
4 slices of mozzarella (or one 120g ball, sliced)

Tomato and basil salad
200g cherry tomatoes, quartered
2 spring onions, chopped
Small handful of fresh basil leaves
1 tsp balsamic vinegar
1 tsp olive oil

To serve
4 tsp reduced-fat basil pesto
Fresh basil leaves

Mix the garlic powder, mixed herbs, onion powder, olive oil, balsamic vinegar and black pepper in a bowl. Add the chicken to the mixture, coat thoroughly and marinate for at least 30 minutes.

While the chicken is marinating, make the tomato and basil salad. Mix all the ingredients and place in the fridge.

Heat a barbecue or griddle pan to high and cook the chicken until it's cooked through. Once cooked, place the chicken on a baking tray, top with the mozzarella slices and place under a grill until the cheese starts to bubble.

To serve, plate up the chicken breasts with a teaspoon of reduced-fat green pesto on top of each plate, some spoonfuls of the salad and garnish with fresh basil leaves.

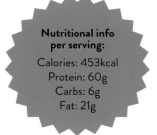

**Nutritional info
per serving:**
Calories: 453kcal
Protein: 60g
Carbs: 6g
Fat: 21g

Prep time: 20 minutes + 30 minutes to marinate
Cook time: 20 minutes
Serves: 3

5 580719 367649

CHEAT'S GREEN CURRY

461 CALORIES per serving

I knew Thai basil was a major flavour in Thai cooking but you don't see it much in other cuisines so I wanted to see if you could make a curry with a classic basil pesto instead of buying a jar of green curry paste only for half of it to go in the bin (green pesto is much more versatile). But I couldn't see that anyone had really given it a go so this was a bit trial-and-error to begin with. Anyway, I think I nailed it cooking for my family – see what you think!

INGREDIENTS

Curry paste
½ onion, roughly chopped
2 tsp minced ginger
2 garlic cloves, crushed
30g low-fat basil pesto
Juice of ½ lime
1 tsp curry powder
2 tbsp water

Curry
1 tbsp coconut oil
1 carrot, sliced
3 spring onions, sliced
1 red pepper, sliced
50g mangetout
500g chicken breasts, sliced
Black pepper
1 tsp brown sugar
400ml light coconut milk
1 tbsp fish sauce
Fresh basil, for garnish

Add all of the ingredients for the curry paste to a blender and blitz.

Heat a wok or large frying pan on a high heat, add the coconut oil and all the vegetables and fry until they start to lightly char. Add the chicken slices, season with black pepper and cook until there aren't any visible pink bits – it doesn't need to be fully cooked through at this stage.

Add the curry paste and fry for a further minute.

Reduce the heat to medium and add the brown sugar, coconut milk and fish sauce. Simmer for about 10 minutes until the sauce has reduced to the consistency of cream.

Serve garnished with fresh basil.

Nutritional info per serving:
Calories: 461cal
Protein: 54g
Carbs: 14g
Fat: 21g

Prep time: 10 minutes
Cook time: 15 minutes
Serves: 3

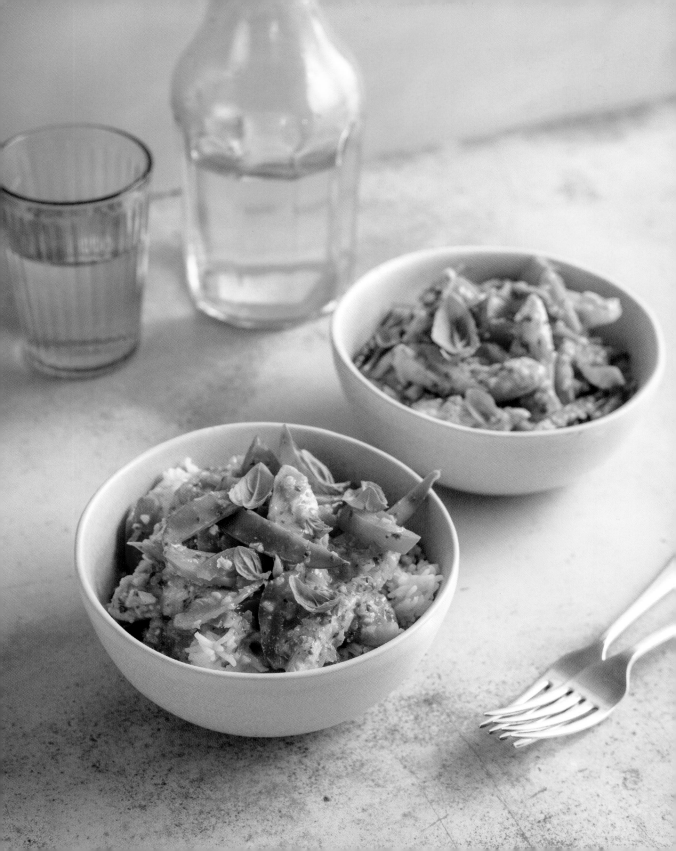

LIGHTER TUSCAN CHICKEN

This is so rich and creamy you'll be amazed to find it comes in at under 400 calories per portion. I've played around with this familiar recipe and come up with a version that's just as tasty and loads healthier. The wine isn't essential in this dish so you could drop it and use extra stock if you prefer.

INGREDIENTS

1 tsp onion powder
1 tsp garlic powder
1 tsp paprika
1 tsp olive oil
1 tbsp water
Black pepper
500g chicken breasts
1 tsp butter
1 red onion, finely chopped
2 garlic cloves, crushed
100g cherry tomatoes, quartered
100ml white wine
30g sun-dried tomato pesto
1 tsp mixed herbs
250ml chicken stock
70ml double cream
30g low-fat cheddar cheese
Handful of fresh basil
100g spinach leaves, washed and trimmed

Mix the onion powder, garlic powder, paprika, olive oil, water and black pepper in a bowl and add the chicken breasts. Get your hands in and make sure the chicken breasts are fully covered in the mixture.

Heat a large frying pan on a medium heat and add the butter. Add the chicken to the pan and fry until brown on all sides. It doesn't need to be fully cooked through at this stage.

Remove the chicken from the pan, set aside and add the onion, garlic and tomatoes and fry until the tomatoes start to break down and the onion begins to brown.

Add the wine and reduce by half. Return the chicken to the pan with the pesto, mixed herbs and chicken stock and simmer for 5–7 minutes.

Add the double cream, cheddar, basil and spinach to the pan and mix through until the spinach wilts.

Nutritional info per serving:
Calories: 374kcal
Protein: 43g
Carbs: 10g
Fat: 18g

Prep time: 10 minutes
Cook time: 30 minutes
Serves: 4

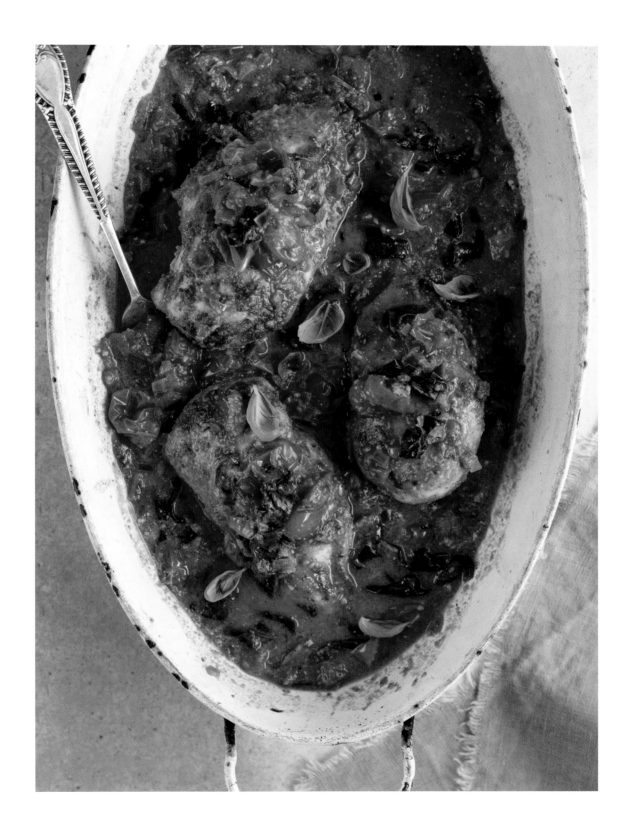

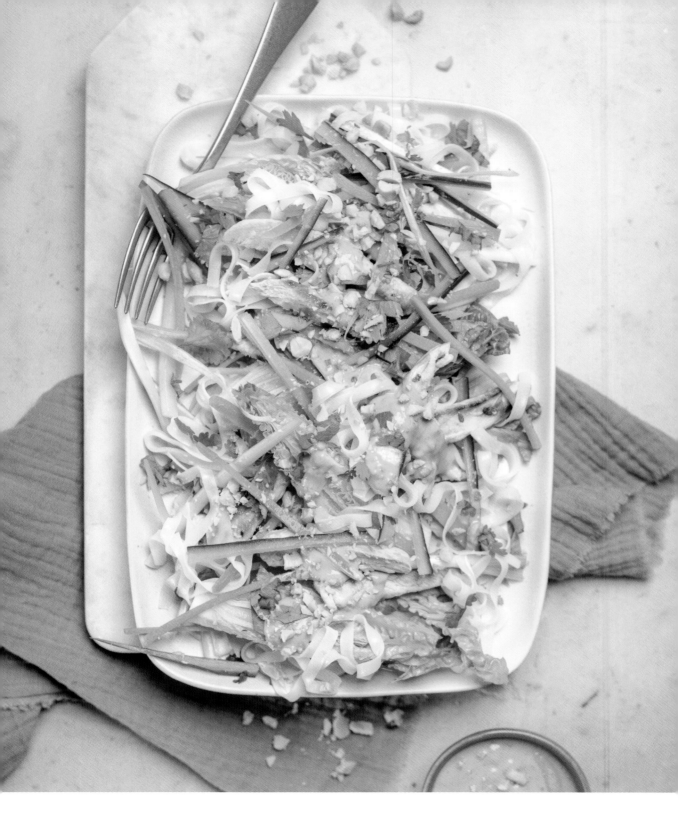

CHICKEN SATAY SALAD

This crisp and crunchy salad combines warm noodles and chicken in a spicy dressing for a delicious lunch or supper. It's easy to make and tastes great at any time of the year.

INGREDIENTS

1 tbsp vegetable or groundnut oil
400g chicken breasts
100g rice noodles (dry weight)
1 large carrot, cut into thin matchsticks
½ small cucumber, cut into matchsticks
4 spring onions, thinly sliced
Handful of fresh coriander, chopped
2 Little Gem lettuces, bases trimmed
60g salted roasted peanuts, roughly
  crushed

Satay dressing
60g crunchy peanut butter
1 tbsp groundnut oil
1 garlic clove, crushed
1 tsp grated ginger
1 tbsp sweet chilli sauce
1 tbsp fish sauce
Juice of 1 lime
1–2 tbsp water (if needed)

Heat the oil in a non-stick frying pan or griddle pan over a medium heat. Add the chicken to the pan and cook for 12–15 minutes, turning halfway through, until golden brown on the outside and cooked right through. Cut into thin slices.

While the chicken is cooking, blitz all the ingredients for the satay dressing in a blender or food processor until smooth. If it's too thick, add a little water to thin it. Transfer to a large bowl and stir in the warm chicken.

Meanwhile, cook the rice noodles according to the directions on the packet. Drain well.

Add the noodles, carrot, cucumber, spring onion and most of the coriander to the chicken together with the lettuce, cut into wedges or separated into leaves. Gently toss everything together until lightly coated.

Divide between four serving plates and sprinkle with the crushed peanuts and remaining coriander. Serve immediately.

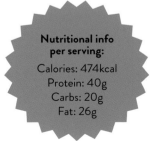

**Nutritional info
per serving:**
Calories: 474kcal
Protein: 40g
Carbs: 20g
Fat: 26g

Prep time: 20 minutes
Cook time: 12–15 minutes
Serves: 4

3 460341 955198

ZA'ATAR CHICKEN KEBABS

401
CALORIES
per serving

Now, I know one of the tenets of this book is that you can find pretty much all the ingredients in your local shop and, at first glance, you may think that za'atar seasoning is going to test that rule. However, it's really gained prominence in recent years and you should find it in most large supermarkets. If you're really struggling to find it, have a quick Google and you can make a passable version of your own with oregano, cumin, etc.

INGREDIENTS

500g chicken breasts, chopped into cubes

Marinade
1 tbsp za'atar seasoning
1 tbsp lemon juice
2 tbsp olive oil
1 tsp honey
½ tsp turmeric
1 tsp Worcestershire sauce
Pinch of chilli flakes
Few grinds of black pepper

Yoghurt dip
150g low-fat natural yoghurt
1 tsp mint sauce
1 garlic clove, finely chopped
1 tbsp lemon juice
Few tsp of finely chopped fresh mint
  and parsley
Few grinds of salt and pepper

Mix the marinade ingredients together and add the chopped chicken breasts. Cover and refrigerate for at least 2 hours.

Mix all the ingredients for the yoghurt dip and set aside.

Heat a barbecue, grill or griddle pan on a medium to high heat. Thread the chicken pieces on to skewers and cook them on both sides until the chicken is cooked through. If using wooden skewers, make sure to soak them in water for 20 minutes before cooking so they don't catch fire.

Serve with a cucumber, tomato, mint and red onion salad, flatbread or rice, and lashings of the yoghurt dip.

**Nutritional info
per serving:**
Calories: 401kcal
Protein: 54g
Carbs: 8g
Fat: 17g

Prep time: 10 minutes +
2 hours to marinate
Cook time: 15 minutes
Serves: 3

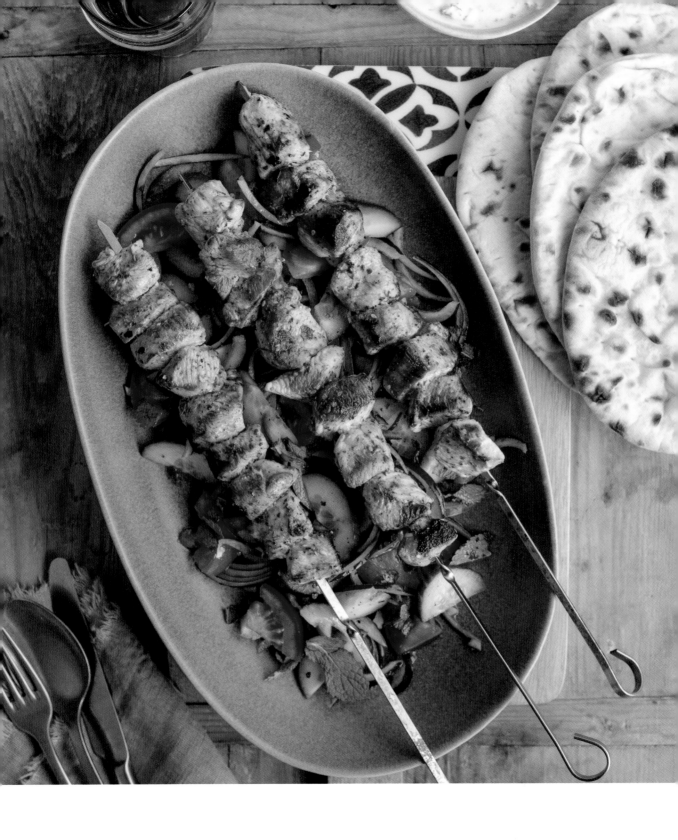

PORK BANH MI

632
CALORIES
per serving

Banh mi is a popular baguette-like sandwich from Vietnam, and pork one of the classic fillings. You might think baguettes aren't traditional Vietnamese fare, but in fact the French introduced them to Vietnam in the mid-nineteenth century. The first time I had a banh mi was on honeymoon in Vancouver. I remember this for two reasons: one, the sandwich was amazing, and two I accidentally dropped a huge dollop of sauce onto my shorts and had to walk around for the rest of the day wearing my lunch. Worth the risk!

INGREDIENTS

Pork
500g pork fillet, cubed
1 tsp brown sugar
1 garlic clove, crushed
1 tsp minced ginger
1 tsp fish sauce
2 tbsp soy sauce
1 tbsp Sriracha

Veg
250g carrots, cut into matchsticks
150g radishes, very finely sliced
2 tbsp rice wine vinegar

To serve
40g light mayonnaise
20g hoisin sauce
3 baguettes
⅓ cucumber, thinly sliced
Handful of fresh coriander

Mix together all the ingredients for the pork and marinate for at least 30 minutes.

While the pork is marinating, mix the carrot and radish with the rice vinegar to gently pickle.

Mix the mayo and hoisin sauce to make a delicious spread.

To cook the pork, thread the cubes on to skewers (soaked for 20 minutes in water if they are wooden) and cook for around 15 minutes on a barbecue or under a grill until cooked through.

Once the pork is cooked, build your sandwich. Start with a spread of the hoisin mayo, then add the sliced cucumber, the pork, some of the vegetables and top with fresh coriander.

Nutritional info
per serving:
Calories: 632kcal
Protein: 48g
Carbs: 74g
Fat: 16g

Prep time: 40 minutes
Cook time: 15 minutes
Serves: 3

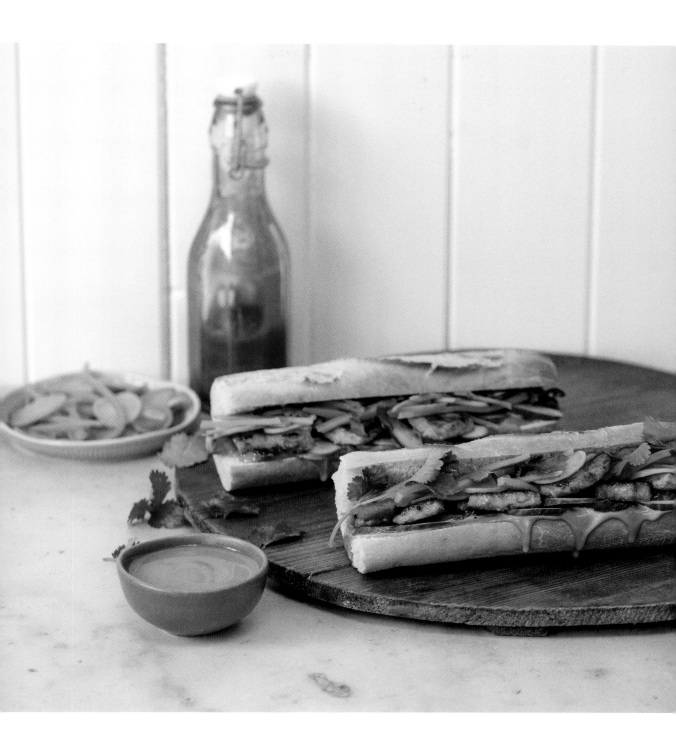

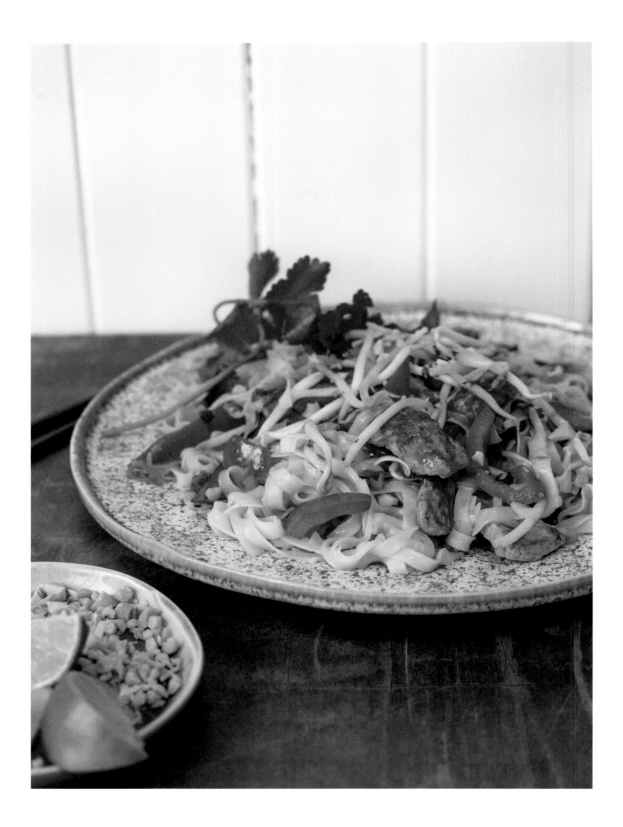

SPICY THAI PORK NOODLES

A delicious Thai street food recipe that whisks you off to the hustle and bustle of a busy Bangkok night market. Quick to prepare and make, this is a great choice midweek. Sriracha seasoning may prove a bit tricky to find, so if you can't get any just use chilli flakes and a bit of extra garlic and ginger.

INGREDIENTS

200g pad Thai rice noodles (dry weight)
1 tbsp sesame oil
500g pork loin, sliced into strips
1 red pepper, sliced
4 spring onions, chopped
2 garlic cloves, crushed
2 tsp minced ginger
200g bean sprouts
30g peanuts, chopped, for garnish
Handful of fresh coriander, for garnish

Sauce
1 tbsp honey
1 tbsp water
1 tsp fish sauce
1 tbsp reduced-salt soy sauce
½ tsp Sriracha

Cook the noodles according to the packet instructions.

Make the sauce by mixing all the ingredients together and set aside.

Heat the sesame oil in a large pan or wok on a high heat and fry the pork until golden brown. Remove from the pan and set aside.

Fry the pepper, spring onion, garlic and ginger for a few minutes, then add the bean sprouts and cook for a few more minutes. Return the pork to the pan along with the drained noodles and sauce.

Serve the noodles garnished with peanuts and some fresh coriander.

Prep time: 10 minutes
Cook time: 10 minutes
Serves: 3

9 350643 435389

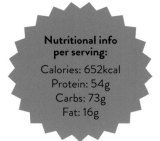

Nutritional info per serving:
Calories: 652kcal
Protein: 54g
Carbs: 73g
Fat: 16g

MEXICAN SAUSAGE WRAPS

247 CALORIES per wrap

I'll be honest – I am not sure if Mexican sausages are a real thing. Or at least they're probably not like these, which are more of kofte than sausage really. But, listen, do we really care when they taste this good? The chorizo gives the recipe that delicious smokey flavour and when you add the lime, salsa, coriander and avocado, you really have a taste of Mexico on your plate. If you can't find reduced-fat chorizo in your supermarket, just use the full-fat kind but be aware this will increase the total calories for the dish.

INGREDIENTS

Sausages
100g reduced-fat chorizo, chopped
500g 5%-fat pork mince
1 tbsp fajita spice mix
2 garlic cloves, chopped
10g tomato purée
1 tbsp olive oil

The rest
1 red onion, chopped
Squeeze of lime or lemon juice
Water, for soaking
8 wholemeal wraps
Salsa
Lime wedges
Sliced avocado
Fresh coriander

Here's a great tip to remove the harsh taste of onions and make them more enjoyable in salads or in tacos, as in this recipe. Simply soak the chopped red onion in a bowl with just enough water to cover and a squeeze of lime or lemon juice for 15 minutes. When you're ready to eat them, drain the water away and serve.

Throw the chorizo into a blender and blitz until it's the same kind of consistency as mince. Add the pork mince, fajita spice, garlic and tomato purée to the blender and blitz again so it's all mixed through.

Form the mixture into about eight sausage shapes. Heat the olive oil in a frying pan on a medium heat and gently fry the sausages for about 10–15 minutes until cooked through.

Serve in a wrap with some salsa, a little sour cream, chopped onion, the lime wedges and avocado, with coriander for garnish.

Nutritional info per wrap:
Calories: 247kcal
Protein: 19g
Carbs: 18g
Fat: 11g

Prep time: 15 minutes
Cook time: 10–15 minutes
Makes: 8 wraps

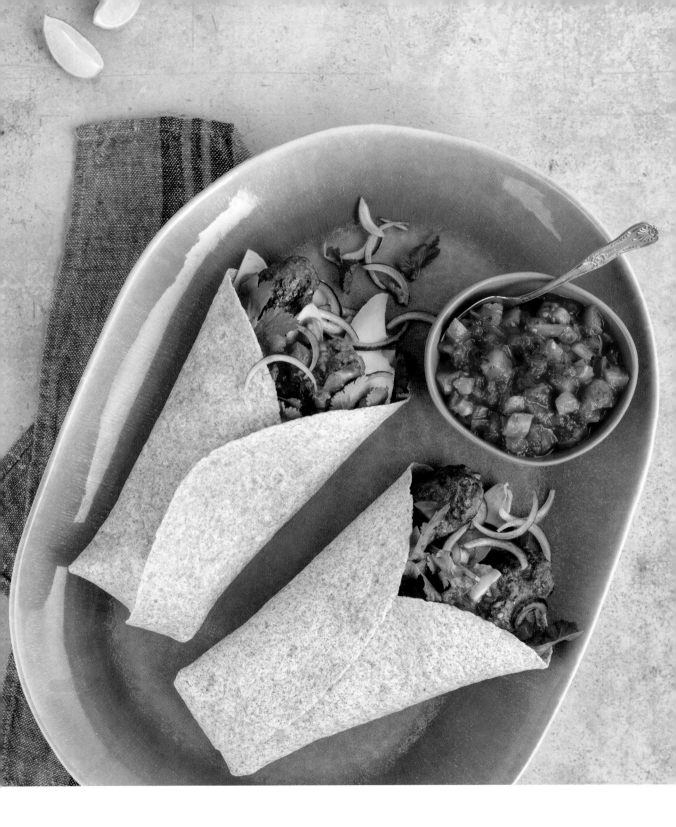

SWEET POTATO *and* CHORIZO SOUP

320
CALORIES
per serving

When you combine the high-fibre, carbohydrate goodness of sweet potato with amazing fiery chorizo, you're on to a winner. This is a contender for the best soup you'll ever make. There, I said it. Try it and see if you disagree.

INGREDIENTS

1 tbsp olive oil
2 red onions, chopped
2 garlic cloves, chopped
2 carrots, chopped
2 peppers (any colour), chopped
200g chorizo, chopped
1 tsp curry powder
1 tsp chilli powder
800g sweet potato, chopped
2 litres stock (any kind)
Salt and pepper

Heat a large, deep pan on a low heat with the olive oil and add the onion, garlic, carrots, peppers, chorizo and the curry and chilli powders. Fry gently for 10 minutes.

Once cooked, add the sweet potato, stock and salt and pepper and simmer for 15 minutes.

Blend everything then serve. Delicious!

Nutritional info per serving:
Calories: 320kcal
Protein: 12g
Carbs: 41g
Fat: 12g

Prep time: 10 minutes
Cook time: 25 minutes
Serves: 6

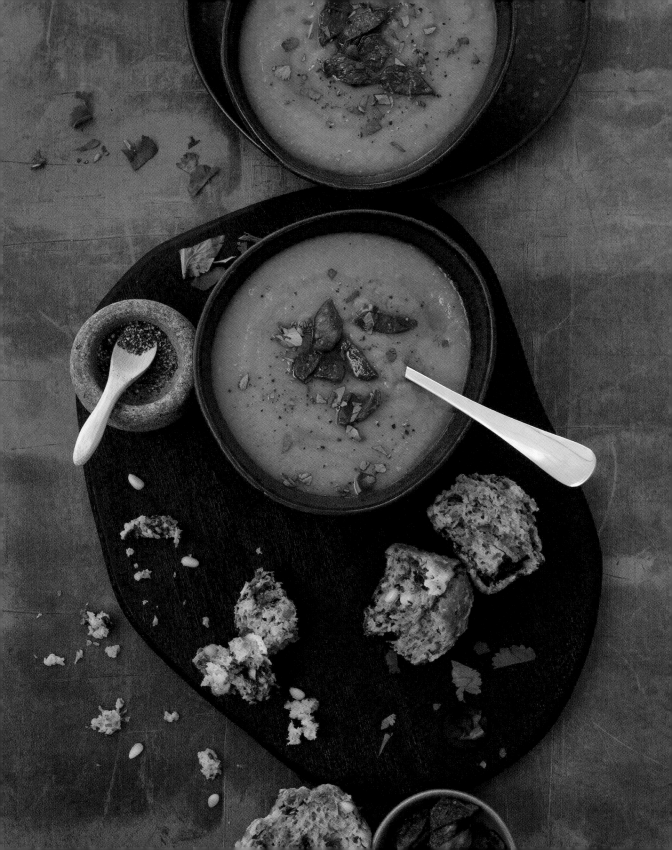

SPANISH TORTILLA WEDGES

557 CALORIES per serving

This healthy Spanish omelette tastes good served hot, warm or at room temperature. It's easy to make and perfect for a light supper, packed lunch or picnic as well as breakfasts and brunches. If you want to go super-authentic, substitute manchego cheese for the cheddar.

INGREDIENTS

3 tbsp olive oil
1 large onion, chopped
2 garlic cloves crushed
500g potatoes, peeled and diced
1 red pepper, diced
100g chorizo, diced
Pinch of chilli flakes
Pinch of smoked paprika
8 medium free-range eggs
Few sprigs of fresh flat-leaf parsley, finely chopped
100g grated low-fat cheddar cheese
Salt and pepper

Heat the oil in a large frying pan set over a low to medium heat. Add the onion, garlic and potato and cook, stirring occasionally, for 10 minutes, or until tender. Stir in the red pepper and chorizo and cook for 4–5 minutes, or until the red pepper is tender and the chorizo sizzles, releases its oil and starts to crisp up. Stir in the chilli flakes and smoked paprika.

Meanwhile, beat the eggs in a large bowl and stir in the parsley and most of the grated cheese. Season lightly with salt and pepper.

Pour the egg mixture into the pan, tilting it to spread it out evenly, and reduce the heat to low. Cook gently for 8 minutes, or until set and golden-brown underneath. Sprinkle the remaining cheese over the top.

Pop the pan under a preheated hot grill for 2–3 minutes until the top of the tortilla is set, puffy and golden brown.

Slide the tortilla out of the pan on to a plate or wooden board and cut into wedges. Serve it hot, lukewarm or cold.

Nutritional info per serving:
Calories: 557kcal
Protein: 31g
Carbs: 25g
Fat: 37g

Prep time: 15 minutes
Cook time: 25–30 minutes
Serves: 4

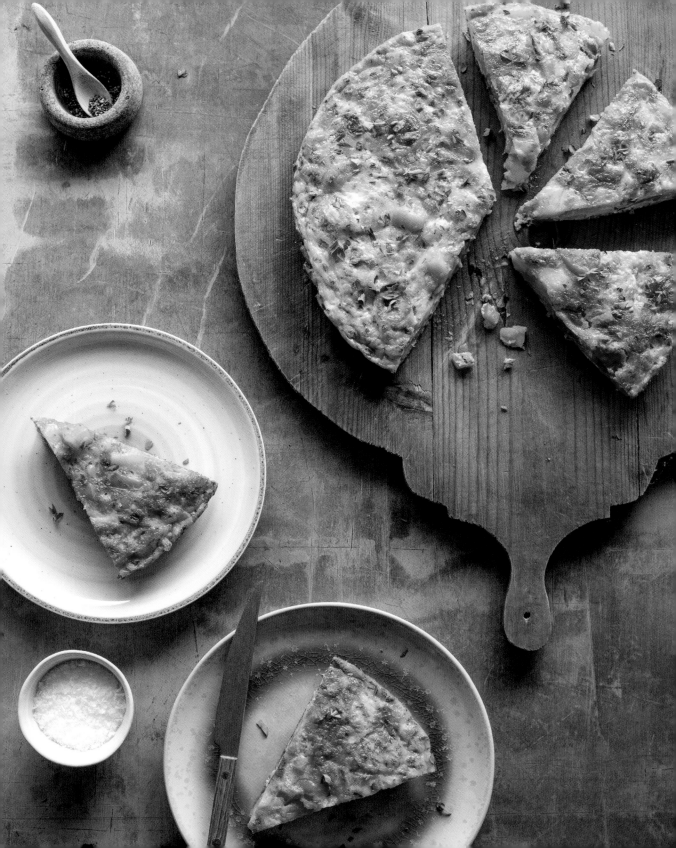

CULLEN SKINK

291
CALORIES
per serving

Cullen skink hails from the small coastal village of Cullen, which is about a 20-minute drive from where I grew up as a kid. This recipe is based on the one my dad has always used. He says it was passed on to him by an ex-colleague's mum, who got it from a very old cookbook, so I'd like to think it's been tried and tested. It's quite filling, so for some it's a meal in itself.

INGREDIENTS

1kg potatoes, peeled and chopped into small chunks
1 onion, finely chopped
500ml semi-skimmed milk
250ml water
500g smoked, skinned haddock fillets
20g butter
170ml evaporated milk
Fresh parsley, chopped, for garnish
Salt and pepper

Add the potato, onion, milk and water to a large soup pan and season with salt and pepper.

Place the haddock fillets flat on top and dot with a few knobs of butter.

Cover the pan and simmer on a low heat for about 20 minutes or until the potatoes are cooked through.

Add the evaporated milk and immediately blend to your desired consistency – some like it smooth, others quite lumpy. Season to taste and serve with chopped parsley.

Nutritional info per serving:
Calories: 291kcal
Protein 20g
Carbs 37g
Fat 7g

Prep time: 10 minutes
Cook time: 20 minutes
Serves: 6

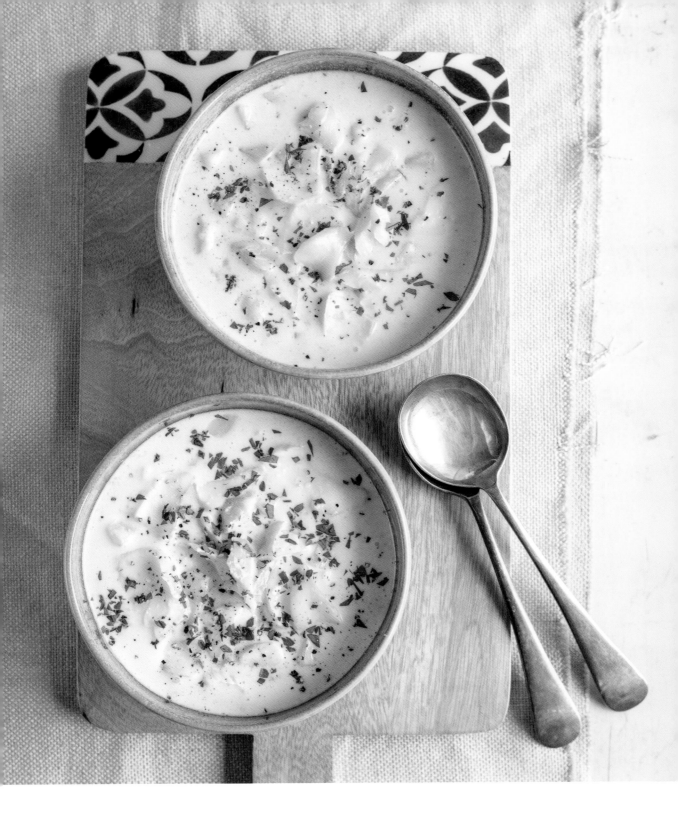

FUNCY FISH FINGER SANDWICH

516 CALORIES per roll

'Funcy' is a NE Scotland way of saying 'fancy', of course. I need to doff my hat to one of my favourite local pubs up here in Aberdeenshire – The Boat Inn in Aboyne – for the inspiration behind this recipe. I was there for lunch with my daughter after her swimming lesson one day and I went for their fish sub. It was delicious so I decided to give it a go myself. Their fish was deep-fried so I've come up with a much lighter option to keep the calories down without compromising on crunch or flavour. If you don't have an air fryer, you should get one. Alternatively, you could pan-fry the goujons or oven bake them, but an air fryer will give you the crunchy coating on the fish that most closely resembles deep-fat frying.

INGREDIENTS

1 red onion, sliced into rings
2 eggs
2 tbsp plain flour
80g cornflakes, crushed
500g white fish fillets, such as haddock, cut into goujons
Cooking spray
4 white rolls (soft, crusty, your pick)
Tartare sauce
3 tomatoes, sliced
Handful of gherkins, sliced
Fresh parsley, roughly chopped

Start things off by placing the sliced onion rings in a bowl of cold water and leave them while you prepare the other ingredients. This will help remove their sharp, bitter tang.

Crack both eggs into a bowl and whisk and set aside. Get another bowl and add the flour, then get a large plate and empty the crushed cornflakes on to it.

Dredge each fish goujon in the flour, then dunk into the egg, then coat with crushed cornflakes and set aside.

Give each of the goujons a light spray with some olive oil or low-cal cooking spray, then place in an air fryer for 10 minutes at 200°C and turn midway through. If you don't have an air fryer you can pan-fry until cooked through instead.

To prepare the rolls, spread each one with some tartare sauce, remove the onions from the water and add some of them along with the tomatoes and gherkins. Place a few fish goujons in each roll and scatter with fresh parsley.

Nutritional info per roll:
Calories: 516kcal
Protein: 34g
Carbs: 59g
Fat: 16g

Prep time: 20 minutes
Cook time: 10 minutes
Makes: 4 rolls

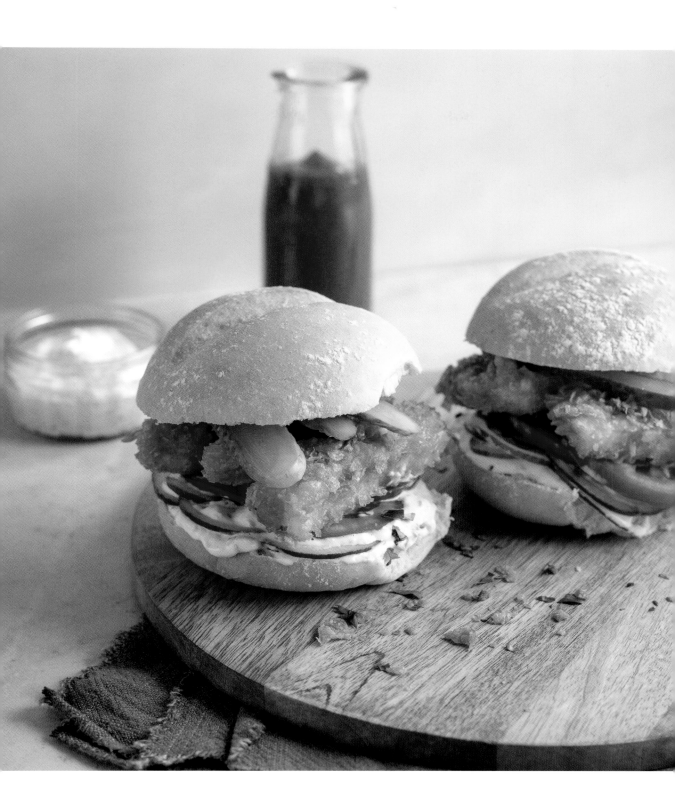

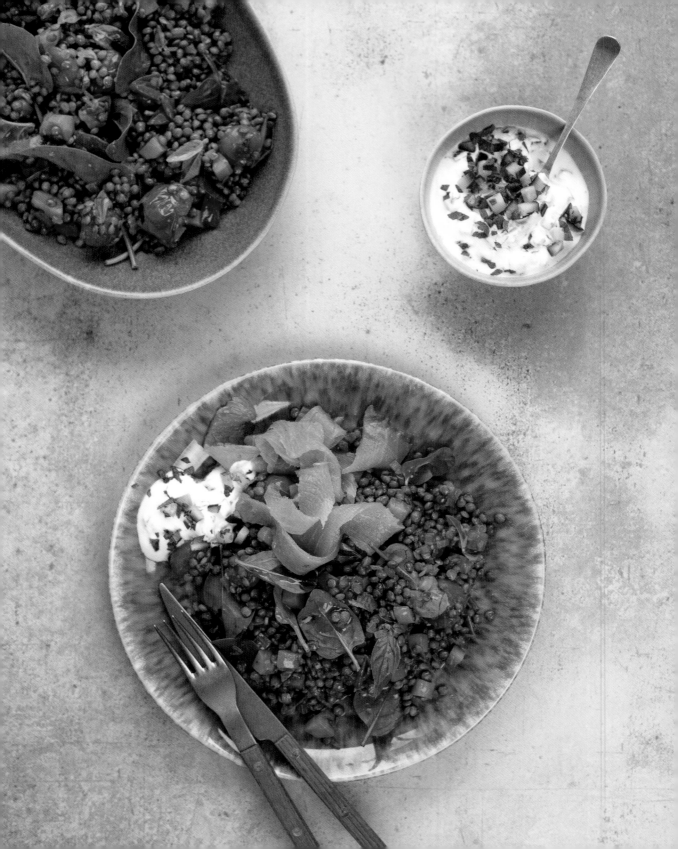

LENTIL *and* SMOKED SALMON SALAD

305 CALORIES per serving

Lentils are a really good and economical source of plant protein plus they taste delicious, too, adding a distinctive earthy flavour to salads. You can make this dish even simpler and quicker by not cooking the onion, garlic and carrots, and just toss the cooked lentils in some vinaigrette with the tomatoes, spinach and basil. Don't be tempted to use small red lentils to make this salad. They go soft and mushy when they are cooked. You need the small green, brown or even black lentils that keep their shape.

INGREDIENTS

250g brown or green lentils (dry weight)
1 tbsp olive oil
1 onion, finely chopped
2 large carrots, diced
2 garlic cloves, crushed
400g cherry tomatoes
150g baby spinach leaves
Juice of 1 lemon
Few drops of balsamic vinegar
Handful of fresh basil leaves
200g smoked salmon, thinly sliced
100g tzatziki
Lemon wedges
Salt and pepper

Put the lentils in a saucepan and cover with cold water. Bring to the boil, then reduce the heat and simmer gently for 15–20 minutes, or until they are tender but still have a little bite. Drain and refresh under cold running water.

Meanwhile, heat the oil in a large frying pan set over a low to medium heat. Cook the onion, carrot and garlic for 8–10 minutes, or until they are tender.

Add the tomatoes and cook for 5–10 minutes, stirring occasionally and squashing them down with the back of a wooden spoon so their juices run out. Stir in the lentils and baby spinach leaves and cook for 5 minutes or until the lentils are hot and the spinach wilts. Add the lemon juice, balsamic vinegar and basil. Season to taste with salt and pepper. Remove from the heat and leave for 15 minutes to allow the lentils to cool a little.

When the lentils are lukewarm, divide them between four serving plates. Add the smoked salmon and tzatziki and serve with lemon wedges on the side for squeezing.

Nutritional info per serving:
Calories: 305kcal
Protein: 22g
Carbs: 25g
Fat: 13g

5 859290 540896

Prep time: 15 minutes + 15 minutes to stand
Cook time: 20–25 minutes
Serves: 4

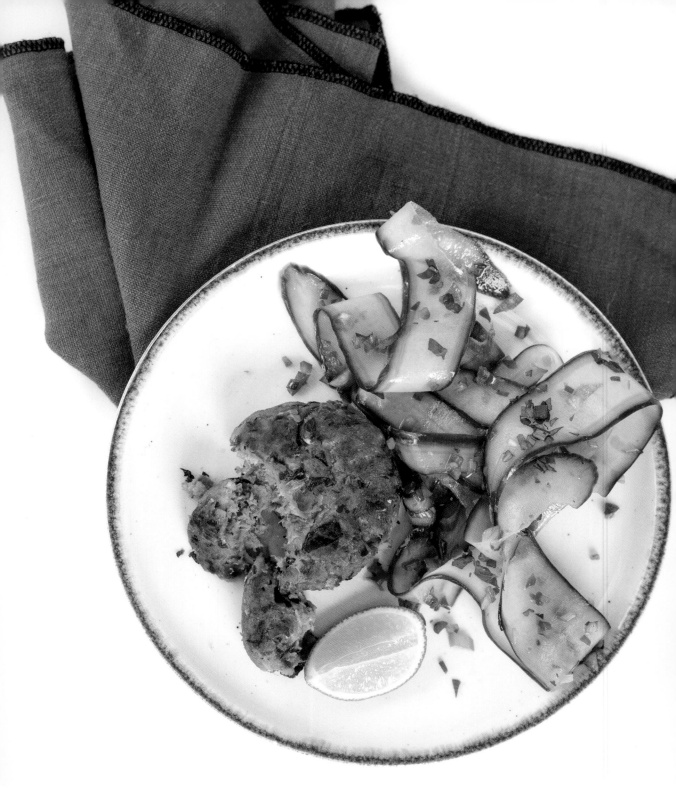

THAI SWEET POTATO FISH CAKES

258
CALORIES
per serving

Fish cakes are delicious, but the problem with most recipes is that they are loaded with cream and butter. This means they're tasty but the fat content is rarely helpful if you're trying to eat healthily. I've got your back – here's a high-protein, low-fat recipe for fish cakes using slow-digesting, high-fibre sweet potatoes.

Now, anyone who has made fish cakes before will know that they require a gentle touch. They're not like a homemade burger, which can be thrown around in a pan. Once you've made your fish cakes, you need to be careful and use a fine touch when you're frying them so they don't fall apart. Treat them with care and you'll be rewarded!

INGREDIENTS

600g sweet potato
2 x 150g tins tuna
4 spring onions, finely chopped
1 tbsp lime juice
2 tsp soy sauce
1 tsp chilli flakes
1 garlic clove, crushed
80g breadcrumbs
Handful of fresh chopped coriander, plus
    extra to garnish
Few grinds of black pepper
2 tbsp coconut or olive oil
Lemon wedges

Peel and chop the sweet potatoes and boil in a large saucepan for around 15 minutes or until cooked.

In a mixing bowl, combine the tuna, spring onion, lime juice, soy sauce, chilli flakes, garlic, breadcrumbs, coriander and pepper.

Once the sweet potato is cooked, drain, mash and spread it out on a plate so it cools quickly.

Once it has cooled enough for you to handle, add it to the bowl with the tuna, getting your hands in and thoroughly combining the mixture. Form into around six fish cake patties and set aside.

Heat the oil in a large frying pan on a low heat and very gently fry the fish cakes for around 4–5 minutes per side. Be careful when turning them to ensure they don't fall apart.

Serve garnished with fresh coriander and some lemon wedges.

Prep time: 15 minutes
Cook time: 30 minutes
Serves: 6

1 189707 379233

Nutritional info
per serving:
Calories: 258kcal
Protein: 22g
Carbs: 29g
Fat: 6g

SPICY SALMON BURGERS

313
CALORIES
per burger

This is one of my favourite recipes: flavoursome, moreish, and ridiculously quick to make. I could eat these all day. A couple of notes on substitutes. Firstly, you can drop the chilli flakes or add more as you need. I find red Thai curry paste isn't that hot, so I usually add extra chilli. If you can't get hold of panko breadcrumbs, or want to make it gluten-free, blitz 50g bread (or GF bread) in a blender to make crumbs, then spread them out on a roasting tray and stick them in the oven at 160°C (140°C fan)/315°F/gas 3 until they start to turn golden brown.

INGREDIENTS

Burgers
400g salmon fillets
1 egg
30g red Thai curry paste
1 garlic clove, crushed
1 tsp minced ginger
1 spring onion
1 tbsp soy sauce
½ tsp chilli flakes
50g panko breadcrumbs

1 tbsp olive oil
Squeeze of lime
Tartar sauce

Add everything for the burgers to a blender and blitz. Remove from the blender and shape with your hands into four burger patties.

Heat the olive oil in a frying pan on a medium heat and cook the burgers for around 4–5 minutes per side.

Serve the burgers with a squeeze of lime and some tartar sauce. Bun and salad leaves optional.

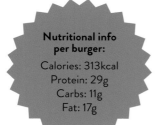

Nutritional info per burger:
Calories: 313kcal
Protein: 29g
Carbs: 11g
Fat: 17g

Prep time: 10 minutes
Cook time: 10 minutes
Makes: 4 burgers

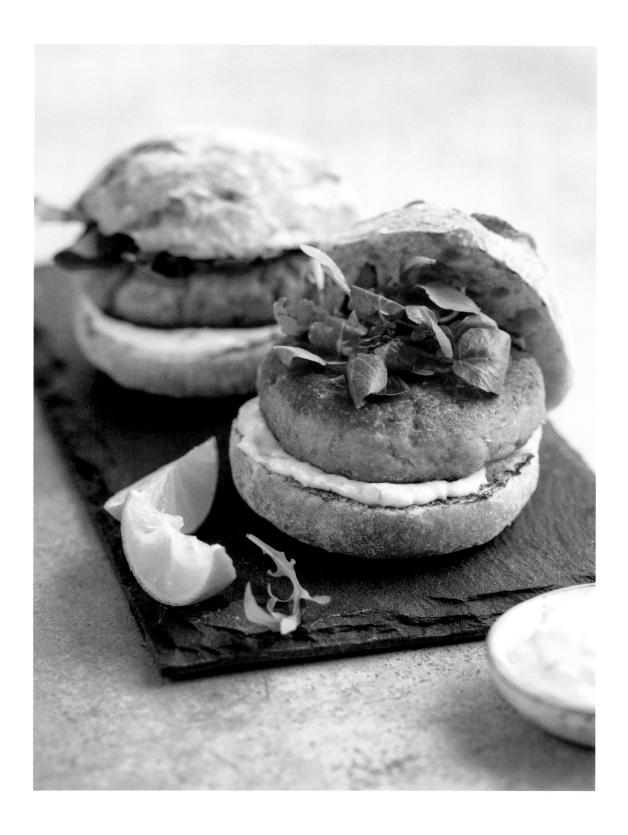

THAI SALMON FOIL PACKETS

455 CALORIES per serving

This easy-to-prepare dish is really something to look forward to – it's healthy, fresh, mouth-watering! Don't like salmon? Just swap it for a different fatty fish such as sea bass or trout and you're good to go. You could also serve with rice or mashed sweet potatoes.

INGREDIENTS

1 garlic clove, finely chopped
1 tsp finely chopped ginger
3 tbsp reduced-salt soy sauce
1 tbsp brown sugar (or sugar substitute for
   lighter version)
1 tsp turmeric
1 tsp sesame oil
2 tbsp lime juice (pretty much the juice of
   1 lime)
2 salmon fillets (around 150g each)
4 spring onions, thinly sliced
1 carrot, thinly sliced
¼ courgette, thinly sliced
200ml chicken stock
100g raw couscous
Fresh coriander

Mix together the garlic, ginger, soy sauce, brown sugar, turmeric, sesame oil and lime juice until well combined.

Marinate the salmon for 30 minutes in the mixture.

Preheat the oven to 200°C (180°C fan)/400°F/gas 6.

Heat a non-stick pan to a high temperature, remove the salmon from the marinade and sear it until it is golden on both sides – around 5 minutes per side. (Note, if you are in a hurry, you can skip this step and add around 10 minutes of baking time, but this step makes it a bit more crunchy.)

Cut out two 30cm foil squares and place half the spring onion, the carrot and courgette on the bottom of each one. Top each with a salmon fillet and start folding to make a packet, adding the remaining marinade and then closing the foil. Place the packets on a baking tray and bake for 20 minutes.

Heat the chicken stock until boiling, cover the couscous with it and let it rest while the salmon is baking. About 5 minutes before removing the salmon from the oven, fluff up the couscous with a fork.

Take the salmon and veggies out of the foil packets and serve them over the couscous topped with the remaining spring onion and fresh coriander.

Nutritional info per serving:
Calories: 455kcal
Protein: 29g
Carbs: 51g
Fat: 15g

Prep time: 35 minutes
Cook time: 30 minutes
Serves: 2

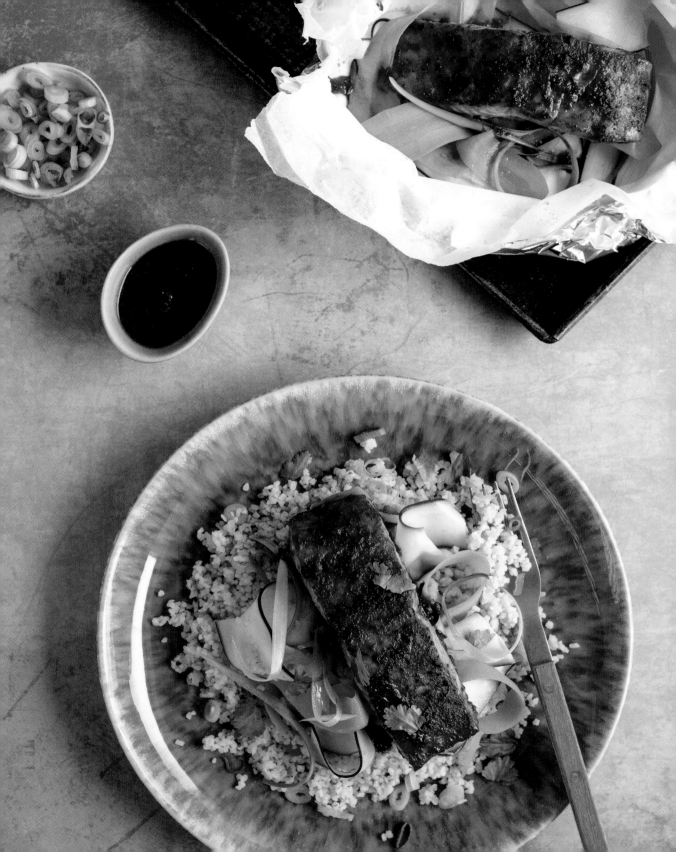

TUNA SALAD PITA POCKETS

446 CALORIES per serving

The filling for this satisfying light lunch is loosely based on the classic French salade niçoise. The delicious combination of eggs and tuna with wholewheat pita delivers a hefty serving of protein. For a lower carb option, try serving this as a salad without the pita. At the other end of the carb spectrum, it's also great with some crusty bread. Or you can leave the tuna chunks whole and mix in some cooked baby new potatoes or pasta shapes.

INGREDIENTS

115g fine green beans, trimmed
4 medium free-range eggs
2 x 150g tins tuna in spring water, drained
Small bunch of spring onions, thinly sliced
1 red or yellow pepper, diced
½ small cucumber, diced
12 cherry tomatoes, quartered
8 juicy black olives, stoned and sliced
1 Little Gem lettuce, chopped
4 large wholewheat pita breads
Few grinds of black pepper

Lemony mayo
4 tbsp light mayonnaise
4 tbsp 0%-fat Greek yoghurt
Squeeze of lemon juice
Few fresh chives, snipped

Make the lemony mayo: put all the ingredients in a bowl and mix well.

Cook the green beans in a saucepan of salted boiling water for 3–4 minutes, or until they beans are just tender but retain a little bite. They should be slightly crisp. Drain and rinse in a colander under cold running water. Pat dry with kitchen paper and cut them in half.

Meanwhile, boil the eggs in a pan of water for 8 minutes. Remove with a slotted spoon and plunge them into a bowl of cold water. Leave until they are completely cold, then peel and chop them.

Mash the tuna with a fork and add to the lemony mayo with the spring onions and some freshly ground black pepper. Gently stir in the diced pepper, green beans, cucumber, tomatoes, olives, lettuce and eggs.

If wished, toast the pita breads; otherwise use them untoasted and cold. Make a slit down the long side of each one and carefully open it up to make a pocket for the filling. Fill with the tuna mayo mixture.

Nutritional info per serving:
Calories: 446kcal
Protein: 47g
Carbs: 33g
Fat: 14g

Prep time: 15 minutes
Cook time: 8 minutes
Serves: 4

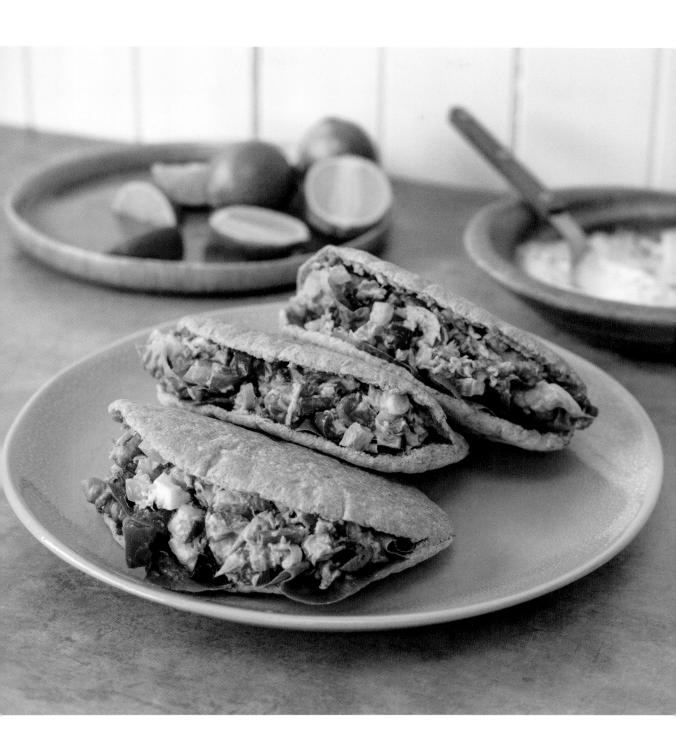

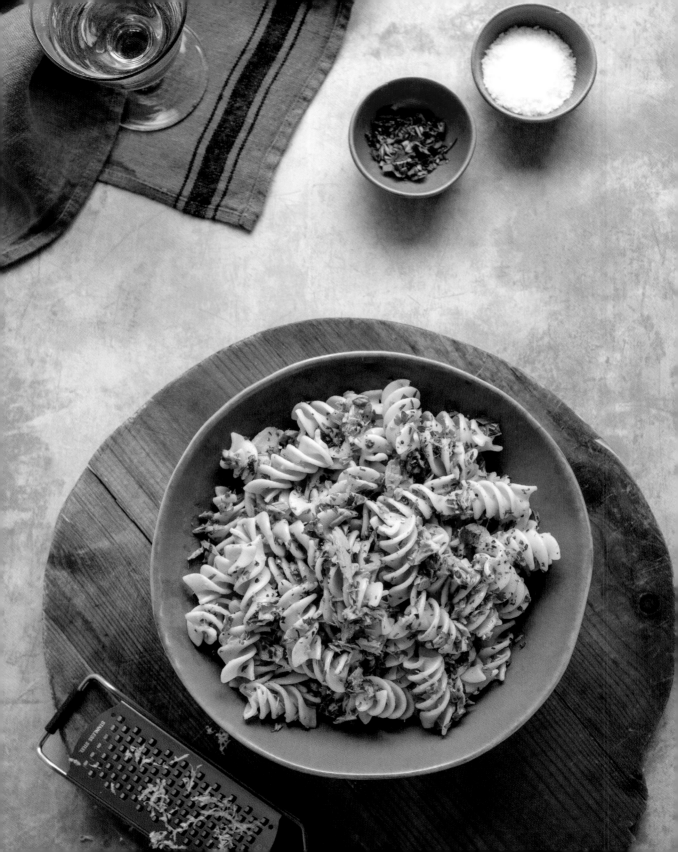

ZINGY TUNA PASTA

466 CALORIES per serving

This is a fresh little recipe for summer that would work well in a lunchbox or served as a side dish at a barbecue. It's incredibly easy to make – prep is a cinch and you can scale this up or down. As always, you can decide if you want to go heavier on the chilli flakes for an extra kick but I think half a teaspoon gives it enough pizazz.

INGREDIENTS

25ml olive oil, plus extra for drizzling
1 red onion, finely chopped
2 garlic cloves, finely chopped
2 tins tuna
½ tsp chilli flakes
½ tsp oregano
Pinch of salt and pepper
Handful of fresh parsley, roughly chopped
Juice of 1 lemon
Zest of ½ lemon
200g pasta (dry weight)

Heat the olive oil in a large pan on a medium heat and fry the onion until it starts to turn golden. Add the garlic and fry for a further 30 seconds.

Add the tuna, chilli flakes, oregano, salt and pepper and fry for a few more minutes.

Add the parsley, lemon juice and zest, mix through and serve with the pasta and a little more olive oil drizzled on top.

Prep time: 5 minutes
Cook time: 10 minutes
Serves: 3

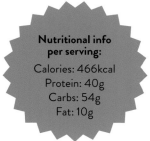

Nutritional info per serving:
Calories: 466kcal
Protein: 40g
Carbs: 54g
Fat: 10g

HALLOUMI SOUVLAKI

705
CALORIES
per serving

You don't have to make a traditional Greek souvlaki with grilled meat – halloumi works brilliantly as an alternative. It's easy and delicious and the perfect vegetarian meal when you don't have much time to cook. If you're ravenously hungry, add some fries or roasted potato wedges.

INGREDIENTS

1 tbsp olive oil
500g halloumi, sliced
4 tbsp plain flour
2 tsp dried oregano
4 large wholewheat flatbreads or wraps
200g tzatziki
Few crisp lettuce leaves, eg cos, shredded
4 ripe tomatoes, sliced or coarsely chopped
1 large red onion, thinly sliced
Handful of fresh flat-leaf parsley, chopped
Smoked paprika, for dusting
Salt and pepper

Heat the oil in a large frying pan or ridged griddle pan set over a medium heat. Lightly dust the halloumi with flour. When the pan is hot, cook the halloumi in batches for 2–3 minutes on each side until crisp, golden brown and starting to soften inside. Alternatively, the halloumi tastes fabulous if you cook it over hot coals on a barbecue. Place the slices on the oiled grill and cook for 2 minutes on each side until golden brown. Take care not to overcook or it will become charred and rubbery. Remove from the pan and drain on kitchen paper. Sprinkle with oregano.

Meanwhile, warm the flatbreads in a low oven or on a hot griddle pan. Spread the tzatziki over each one and top with the lettuce, tomato and onion.

Arrange the halloumi on top with potato wedges or fries. Season with salt and pepper, sprinkle with parsley and dust with smoked paprika.

Fold the flatbreads or wraps over and around the filling and roll up in some greaseproof paper or kitchen foil to hold the filling in place. Eat immediately.

Nutritional info per serving:
Calories: 705kcal
Protein: 39g
Carbs: 45g
Fat: 41g

Prep time: 15 minutes
Cook time: 8–12 minutes
Serves: 4

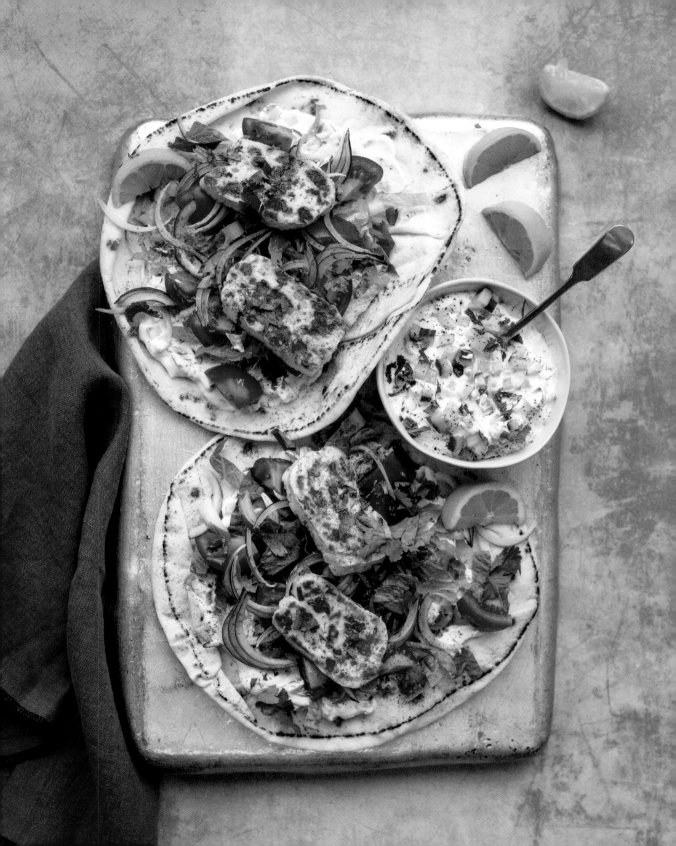

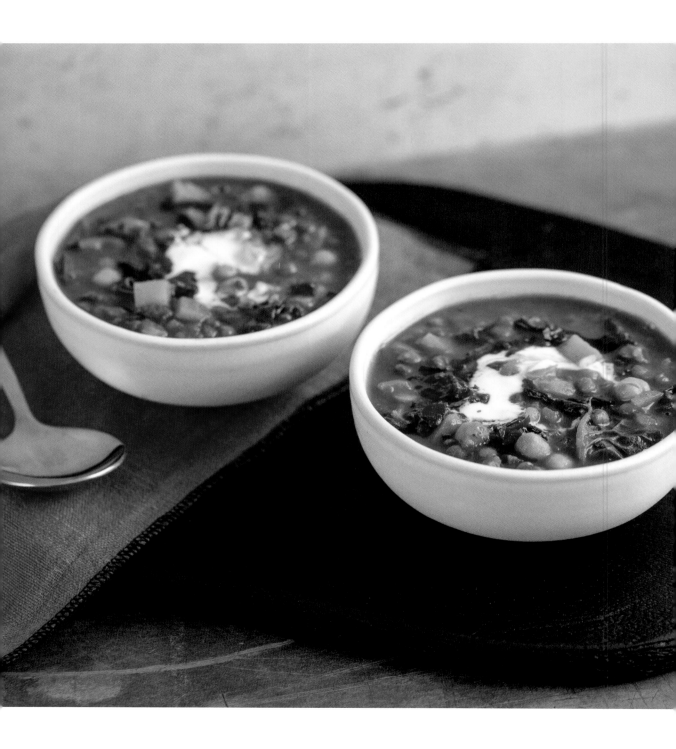

HARIRA
(SPICY MOROCCAN LENTIL SOUP)

470
CALORIES
per serving

VEGGIE

Harira is traditionally eaten after sunset during the month of Ramadan when fasting ends for the day. Sustaining and nutritious, it packs a big punch of vegetable protein and really is a meal in a bowl.

INGREDIENTS

3 tbsp olive oil
2 onions, finely chopped
4 garlic cloves, crushed
2 stalks celery, diced
2 tsp cumin seeds
1 tsp turmeric
½ tsp ground cinnamon
Pinch of chilli flakes
200g brown lentils (dry weight)
2 large potatoes, peeled and cubed
400g tin chopped tomatoes
Bunch of fresh flat-leaf parsley, chopped
1 litre hot vegetable stock
400g tin chickpeas, drained and rinsed
300g spinach leaves, washed, trimmed and
  shredded
Juice of 1 lemon
4 tbsp 0%-fat Greek yoghurt
Salt and pepper
Harissa paste, to serve

Heat the olive oil in a large saucepan set over a medium heat. Cook the onion, garlic and celery, stirring occasionally, for 8–10 minutes or until tender and golden. Stir in the seeds, ground spices and chilli flakes and cook for 1 minute.

Add the lentils and potato and stir gently until they are glistening with oil. Add the tomatoes, parsley and vegetable stock, then bring to the boil.

Reduce the heat and stir in the chickpeas. Simmer gently for 20–25 minutes, or until the lentils are cooked but still hold their shape and the potatoes are tender. Add the spinach and cook for 3–4 minutes until it wilts into the soup. Season to taste with salt and pepper and stir in the lemon juice.

Ladle the soup into bowls and swirl a spoonful of yoghurt and a little harissa paste into each one.

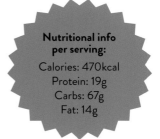

Nutritional info per serving:
Calories: 470kcal
Protein: 19g
Carbs: 67g
Fat: 14g

Prep time: 20 minutes
Cook time: 40–45 minutes
Serves: 4

7 259210 825030

SUMMER BULGUR WHEAT SALAD

385 CALORIES per serving

Bulgur wheat is so delicious and rich in protein and essential minerals. Its mild and nutty flavour and slightly chewy texture goes well with tomatoes, onion, olives and feta in this Mediterranean-style salad. This makes a great packed lunch. Make the salad the day before, chill in the fridge overnight, and put some in a sealed lunchbox to take with you on the go. If you can't find bulgur wheat, you can use quinoa instead.

INGREDIENTS

150g bulgur wheat (dry weight)
240ml boiling water
400g baby plum or cherry tomatoes, quartered
¼ cucumber, cut into chunks
Bunch of spring onions, chopped
2 x 400g tins chickpeas, drained and rinsed
12 black olives, stoned
2 tbsp capers, rinsed and chopped
Handful of fresh coriander or mint, chopped
4 tsp olive oil
Juice of 1 large lemon
200g low-fat feta cheese, crumbled
Seeds of ½ pomegranate, for sprinkling (optional)
Lemon wedges
Salt and pepper

Put the bulgur wheat into a large bowl and pour the boiling water over the top. Stir well and cover with cling film. Leave for 15 minutes, or until the bulgur wheat has absorbed all or most of the water and is tender but still retains some bite. Put the bulgur wheat into a sieve to drain off any excess water.

Transfer the bulgur wheat to a clean bowl and fluff up with a fork. Add the tomato, cucumber, spring onion, chickpeas, olives, capers and herbs. Gently stir in the olive oil and lemon juice, and season to taste with salt and pepper.

Divide between four shallow bowls and crumble the feta over the top. Sprinkle with pomegranate seeds (if using) and serve with some lemon wedges on the side for squeezing.

Nutritional info per serving:
Calories: 385kcal
Protein: 20g
Carbs: 29g
Fat: 21g

Prep time: 15 minutes + 15 minutes to soak
Serves: 4

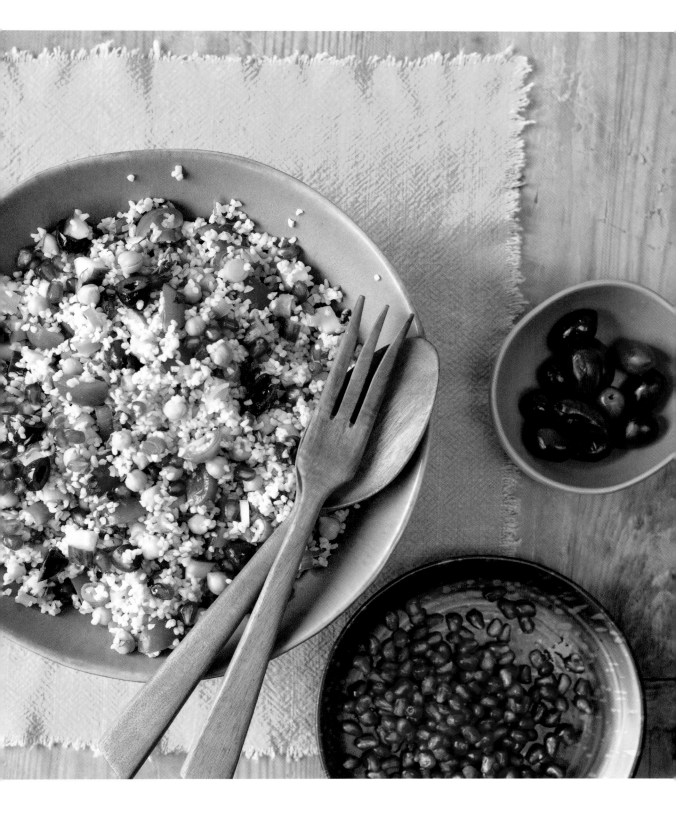

LOU'S LUSH LENTIL CURRY

273 CALORIES per serving

Louise is a pal of mine from school and she's a dab hand at vegetarian cooking. This is one of her epic curry recipes, which is extremely easy to make but ridiculously tasty and less than 300 calories per serving. Not bad, eh? If you've not heard of garam masala before, it's a spice blend that's a base for many Indian dishes and brings flavour and warmth. You can buy it in most supermarkets or grind your own if you're adventurous and want to be super authentic.

To boost the protein content of this meal you could add some beans to keep it vegetarian or it's a delight with chicken.

INGREDIENTS

1 tbsp coconut oil
2 onions, thinly sliced
1 garlic clove, crushed
1 teaspoon minced ginger
200g red lentils, rinsed
500ml vegetable stock
1 tsp ground cumin
1 tsp chilli powder
1 tsp garam masala
400g tin chopped tomatoes
400ml light coconut milk

Heat the coconut oil in a large pan on a medium heat, add the onion and cook for around 10 minutes until softened.

Add the garlic and ginger and cook for a further 2 minutes. Add all the remaining ingredients and mix through.

Reduce the heat to low, cover and simmer for 30 minutes, stirring occasionally.

Remove the pan lid and simmer for a final 15 minutes.

Nutritional info per serving:
Calories: 273kcal
Protein: 12g
Carbs: 36g
Fat: 9g

Prep time: 10 minutes
Cook time: 1 hour
Serves: 5

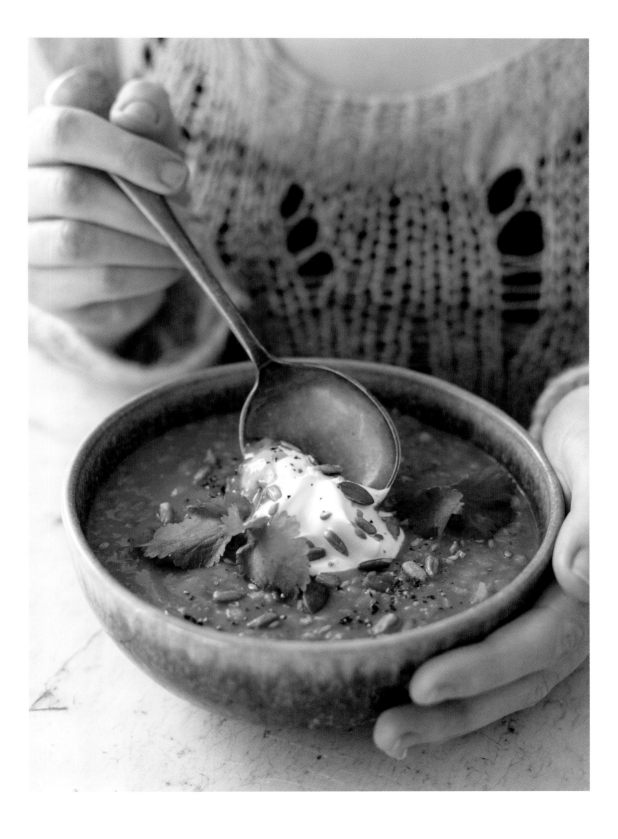

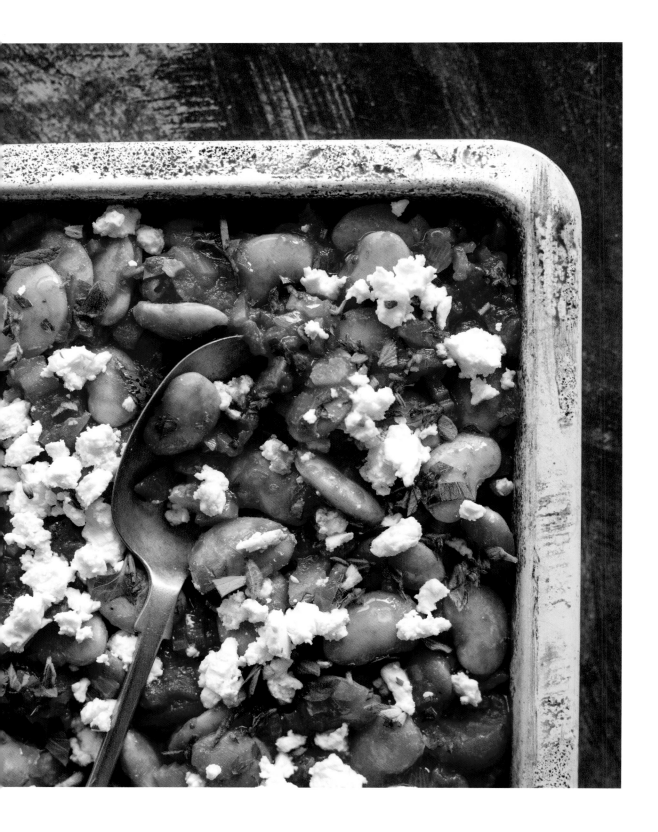

MEDITERRANEAN BAKED BUTTER BEANS

In Greece and the Eastern Mediterranean, this is made with extra-large dried gigantes beans. If you want to be authentic you can buy them online or in delicatessens and specialist stores. However, butter beans work just as well instead. Dried beans are an economical and excellent source of plant protein.

INGREDIENTS

350g dried butter beans (dry weight)
1 tbsp olive oil, plus extra for drizzling
1 onion, finely chopped
2 stalks celery, finely chopped
2 garlic cloves, crushed
2 tbsp tomato purée
2 x 400g tins of plum tomatoes, skinned and coarsely chopped
Leaves stripped from a few fresh oregano sprigs
1 tsp caster sugar
1 tbsp red wine vinegar
Handful of fresh flat-leaf parsley, chopped
150g low-fat feta cheese, crumbled
Salt and pepper

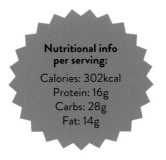

Nutritional info
per serving:

Calories: 302kcal
Protein: 16g
Carbs: 28g
Fat: 14g

Put the butter beans in a large bowl, cover with cold water and leave to soak overnight. The following day, drain the beans, then rinse under cold running water and transfer them to a large saucepan. Cover with plenty of fresh cold water and set over a high heat. When the water boils, reduce to a simmer and cook gently for 45–50 minutes. Do not overcook them – they must keep their shape and should not be soft. Drain in a colander, reserving the cooking liquid.

Preheat the oven to 170°C (150°C fan)/325°F/gas 3.

Heat the olive oil in a saucepan over a medium heat. Cook the onion, celery and garlic, stirring occasionally, for 6–8 minutes, or until tender. Stir in the tomato purée and cook for 1 minute. Add the drained beans, tomatoes, oregano, sugar, vinegar and 400ml of the cooking liquid. This contains starch and adding it to the tomato and bean mixture makes the sauce creamy. Stir well and season with salt and pepper.

Transfer to a large ovenproof baking dish and cover with kitchen foil. Bake for 1–1¼ hours, then remove the foil and cook for 30 minutes, or until the tomato sauce has thickened and the beans are tender.

If the liquid evaporates and the beans seem dry when you remove the foil, moisten with a little hot water.

Leave to cool until the beans reach room temperature. Sprinkle with parsley and crumble the feta over the top. Serve drizzled with olive oil, with some crusty bread on the side.

Prep time: 10 minutes + overnight soaking
Cook time: 2½ –2¾ hours
Serves: 4

MOROCCAN-STYLE CHICKPEA RATATOUILLE

217
CALORIES
per serving

I've put this dish into the light meals section but it's really a bit of a monster. The serving sizes are huge, so you might even want to divide it into six portions instead. Anyway, if your pan is big enough you'll love this recipe. It's very fresh, great for summer eating, can be enjoyed on its own as a 100 per cent vegetarian meal or can be eaten as a side dish to accompany something else. It would work as an epic side dish to the Za'atar Chicken Kebab you can find in this book.

INGREDIENTS

2 tbsp olive oil
2 peppers, roughly chopped
1 onion, roughly chopped
2 courgettes, roughly chopped
1 small aubergine, roughly chopped
2 garlic cloves, chopped
2 tbsp Moroccan seasoning such as
 ras el hanout
2 x 400g tins chopped tomatoes
2 x 400g tins chickpeas, drained and rinsed
Handful of freshly chopped parsley

Heat a large pan on a medium to low heat and add the olive oil. Add all the vegetables, apart from the garlic, and fry for 8–10 minutes.

Add the Moroccan seasoning and the garlic and fry for 1 more minute.

Add the chopped tomatoes and chickpeas, lower the heat to medium and simmer for 10–15 mins.

Garnish with plenty of fresh parsley.

Nutritional info per serving:
Calories: 217kcal
Protein: 10g
Carbs: 24g
Fat: 9g

Prep time: 10 minutes
Cook time: 25 minutes
Serves: 5

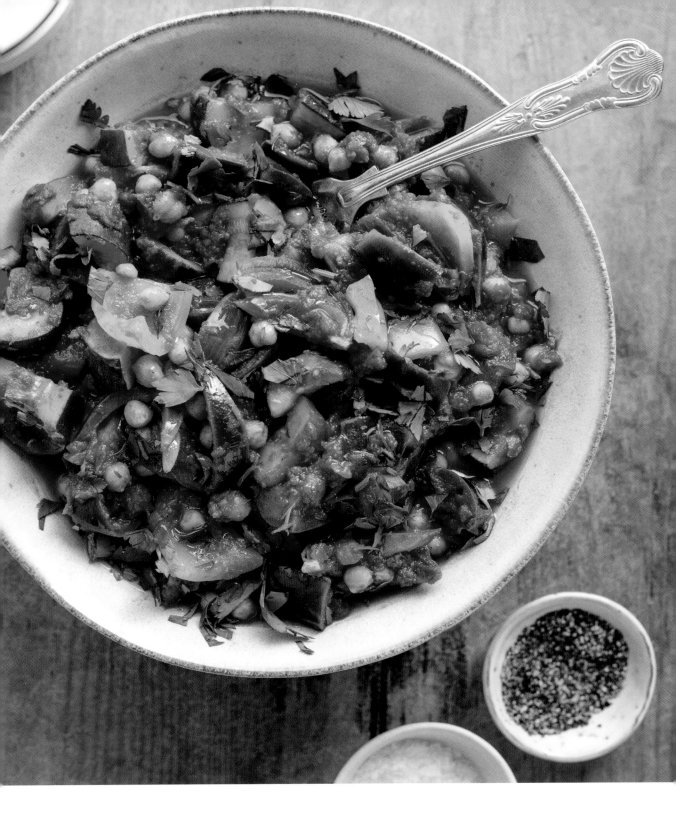

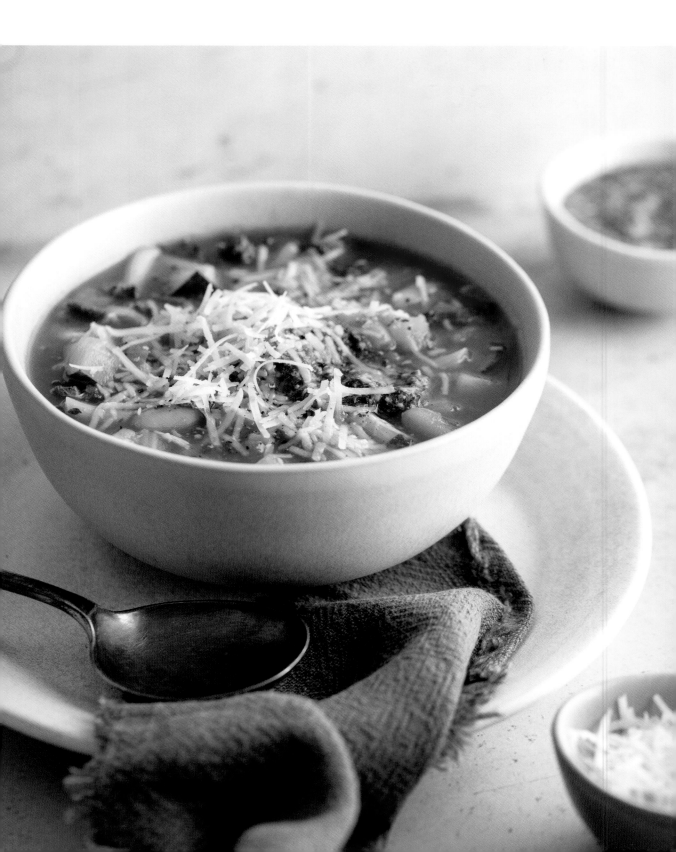

RUSTIC ITALIAN BEAN SOUP

482
CALORIES
per serving

This earthy Italian soup is extremely warming on a cold day. It's easy to make and keeps well stored in the fridge for up to five days. Just reheat it in the microwave or a pan on the hob. As with all soups, this one is easy to scale up if you want more portions.

INGREDIENTS

2 tbsp olive oil
2 onions, finely chopped
3 stalks celery, chopped
2 large carrots, diced
3 garlic cloves, crushed
1.2 litres hot vegetable stock
400g tin chopped tomatoes
1 large potato, peeled and diced
2 courgettes, chopped
400g tin cannellini or borlotti beans, drained and rinsed
Few sprigs of thyme
1 tsp sugar
100g pasta shapes, eg macaroni, ditalini or gomiti (dry weight)
180g spinach, kale or cavolo nero, washed, trimmed and shredded
4 tbsp basil pesto
50g grated Parmesan cheese
Salt and pepper

Heat the oil in a large saucepan set over a low heat and cook the onion, celery, carrot and garlic, stirring occasionally, for 8–10 minutes until softened but not coloured.

Add the stock, tomatoes, potato, courgette, beans, herbs and sugar and bring to the boil. Reduce the heat and simmer gently for 30 minutes. Add the pasta and continue cooking for 10–15 minutes, or until it is tender and al dente.

Stir in the spinach, kale or cavolo nero and cook for 5 minutes, or until the leaves wilt. Season to taste with salt and pepper.

Ladle the soup into four bowls and swirl a spoonful of pesto into each one. Sprinkle with plenty of Parmesan, so it melts into the soup, and serve hot.

Prep time: 20 minutes
Cook time: 1 hour
Serves: 4

3 037248 709089

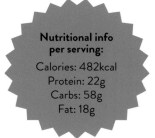

Nutritional info per serving:
Calories: 482kcal
Protein: 22g
Carbs: 58g
Fat: 18g

PART 3
MAIN

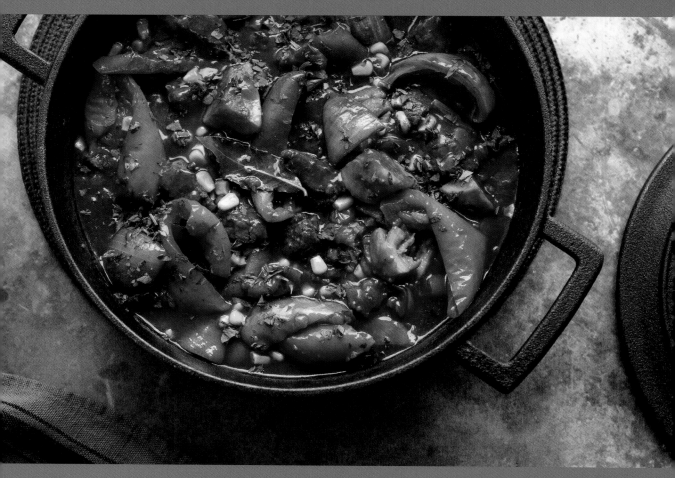

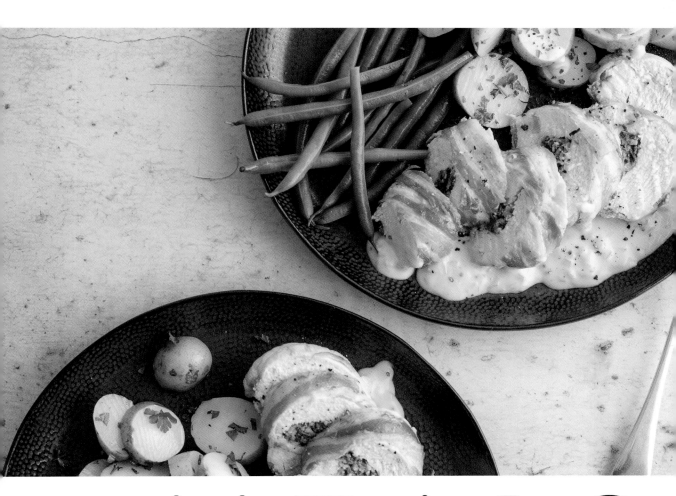

MEALS

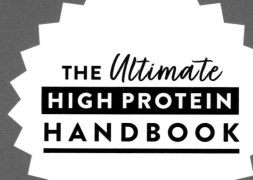

THE *Ultimate*
HIGH PROTEIN
HANDBOOK

THE MAIN MEALS IN THIS SECTION ARE A BIT MORE HEARTY, OFTEN ARE THE BEST ONES TO SCALE FOR MEAL PREP AND ARE THE RECIPES THAT YOU CAN TURN TO WHEN YOU NEED SOMETHING TO PLEASE A CROWD. FOLLOWERS WILL RECOGNISE MORE FROM THIS SECTION INCLUDING THE ALWAYS POPULAR MEXICAN LASAGNE, BRAZILIAN COCONUT CHICKEN CURRY AND ST MARY'S CHICKEN.

SOME OF MY FAVOURITE NEW RECIPES IN THIS SECTION INCLUDE THE CARBONADA CRIOLLA – AN ARGENTINIAN BEEF STEW THAT HAS A DELICIOUS SWEETNESS THANKS TO THE ADDITION OF DRIED APRICOTS AND SWEET POTATO. YES IT SOUND LIKE AN INTERESTING MIX BUT IT'S AN EXTREMELY TASTY ONE AT THAT.

THE CHINESE TAKEAWAY CURRY HAS SAVED ME A GOOD FEW QUID SINCE I CAME UP WITH IT. IT'S MORE OR LESS IDENTICAL IN FLAVOURS TO WHAT YOU'LL GET FROM THE TAKEAWAY BUT A FRACTION OF THE COST, AND CALORIES.

YOU ALSO HAVE TO TRY THE CHORIZO, CHICKEN SAUSAGE AND CHICKPEA STEW RECIPE. IT'S THE ONE THAT IS MOST OFTEN REQUESTED IN THE BAPTIE HOUSEHOLD AND I'VE MADE IT MORE THAN ANY OTHER RECIPE IN THIS BOOK.

BEEF KHEEMA

286 CALORIES per serving

My dad introduced me to this one, although he included a beer in his, which I found a bit odd. So that's been wheeched out and I've added in a few other bits to make it more interesting (sorry dad). Plus I've altered it a bit from the version you may already know and love to make it easier and tastier still. If you're a fan of chillies and Bolognese, then this will hit the spot.

INGREDIENTS

1 tbsp coconut oil
2 onions, chopped
2 garlic cloves, finely chopped
2 tsp minced ginger
20g curry powder
½ tsp chilli powder (optional)
30g tomato purée
1kg 5%-fat beef mince
10 g cornflour
400g tin chopped tomatoes
4 carrots, cubed
1 litre beef stock
150g green peas

Add the coconut oil to a large pan and cook the onion until it starts to turn translucent. Add the garlic and ginger and cook for 30 seconds more. Add the curry powder, chilli powder and tomato purée and cook for another 30 seconds or so.

Add the mince to the pan and brown, breaking it up with a spoon and cooking until no longer pink. Stir through the cornflour.

Add the chopped tomatoes, carrot and stock and simmer for around 20–25 minutes until the sauce has thickened. Add the peas and cook for a further 5 minutes.

Serve with rice and your favourite chutney.

Nutritional info per serving:
Calories: 286kcal
Protein: 36g
Carbs: 13g
Fat: 10g

Prep time: 5 minutes
Cook time: 40 minutes
Serves: 7

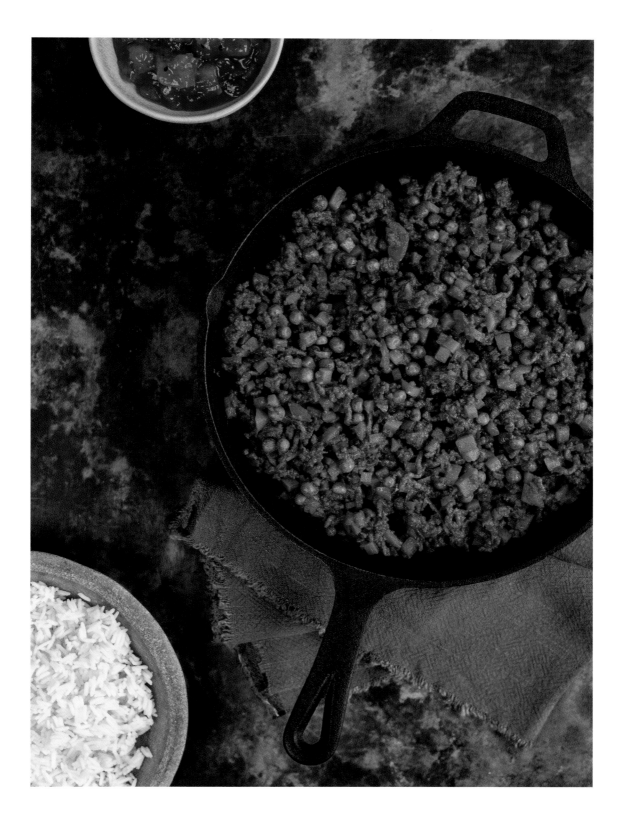

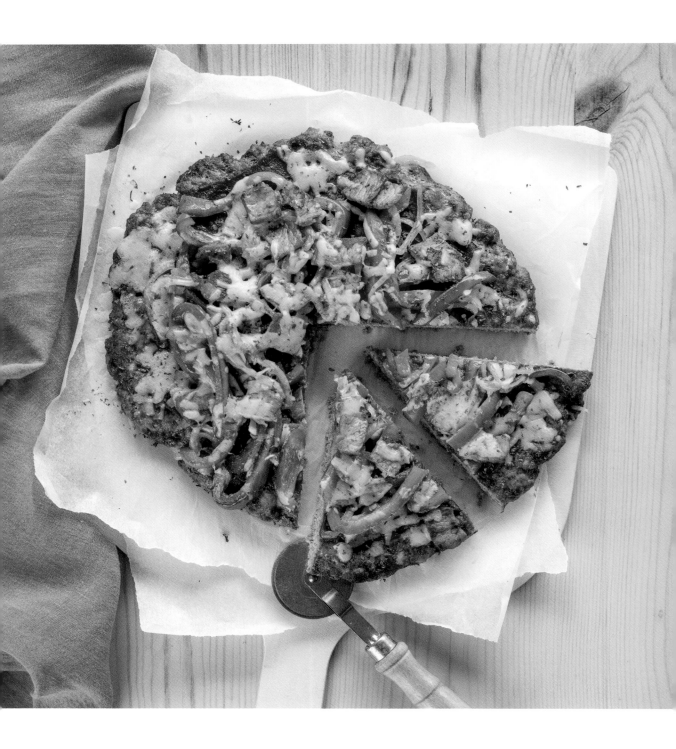

BACON *and* CHEESE-TOPPED MEATZA

If you like meat and pizza, then you're going to love this! Loaded with two different kinds of mince, bacon and topped with cheese, this is a low-carb taste sensation that packs 32g of protein per slice, with only 3g of carbohydrates.

It's really easy to make, you can play around with different toppings, and the whole family will like it. It's also delicious the next day, served cold in a sandwich or cut up in a salad.

INGREDIENTS

500g 5%-fat beef mince
500g 5%-fat pork mince
1 tbsp olive oil
1 onion, chopped
1 red pepper, chopped
1 green pepper, chopped
6 bacon medallions, chopped
2 tbsp tomato purée
1 tbsp mixed herbs
50g low-fat cheddar cheese

Preheat the oven to 230°C (210°C fan)/450°F/gas 8.

To make the base (basically a giant burger), combine the beef and pork mince in a large mixing bowl. Get your hands in and make sure it's all nicely mushed together. Season liberally.

Flatten out the meat mixture on a baking tray so it covers the tray and is around 2–3cm thick, then place the base in the oven for around 15 minutes until the juices run clear and it's cooked through.

While the base is cooking, heat the olive oil in a large frying pan on a medium heat and cook the onion, peppers and bacon for 10 minutes until cooked through. Once done, set aside.

Remove the base from the oven, drain any liquid, if necessary, then cover with the tomato purée and spread it out, just as you would on a normal pizza.

Put the cooked bacon, onion and peppers on top, scatter over the mixed herbs, then sprinkle a thin layer of cheese over everything. Place under a grill for 5 minutes for the cheese to melt before serving.

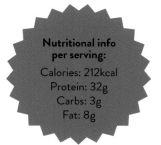

Nutritional info
per serving:
Calories: 212kcal
Protein: 32g
Carbs: 3g
Fat: 8g

Prep time: 20 minutes
Cook time: 25 minutes
Serves: 8

1 499895 459472

BEST DIY BURGER

238 CALORIES per burger

This is a strong basic burger recipe that allows you to add all sorts of flavour combinations to make it taste delicious. For example, I've used fajita seasoning, BBQ, Cajun – or my favourite Montreal Steak Seasoning, – although that's a bit more of a pain to find. Anyway, you've so much flexibility with this one to make something that you'll love.

INGREDIENTS

1 tsp olive oil
1 red onion, very finely chopped
500g 5%-fat beef mince
1 egg
30g oats
1 tbsp of your favourite seasoning (plus ½ tsp salt if your seasoning doesn't have salt as one of the main ingredients)

Heat the olive oil in a pan on a medium heat and fry the onion until it starts to brown. Remove from the heat and allow to cool.

Mix the onion with all the other ingredients and shape the mixture into four burger patties.

Grill, bake or barbecue until the patties are cooked to your desired level of doneness.

Nutritional info per burger:
Calories: 238kcal
Protein: 30g
Carbs: 7g
Fat: 10g

Prep time: 10 minutes
Cook time: 15 minutes
Serves: 4

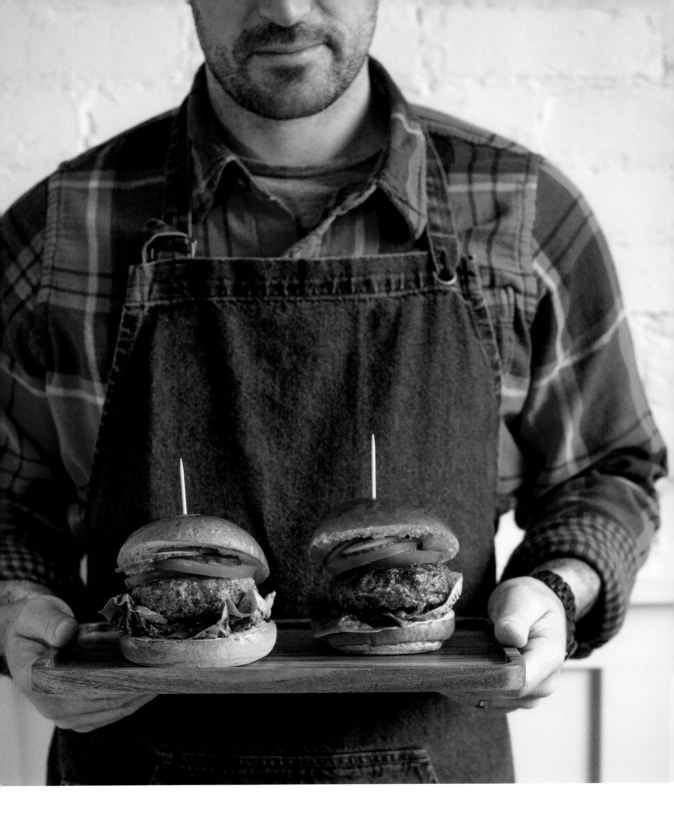

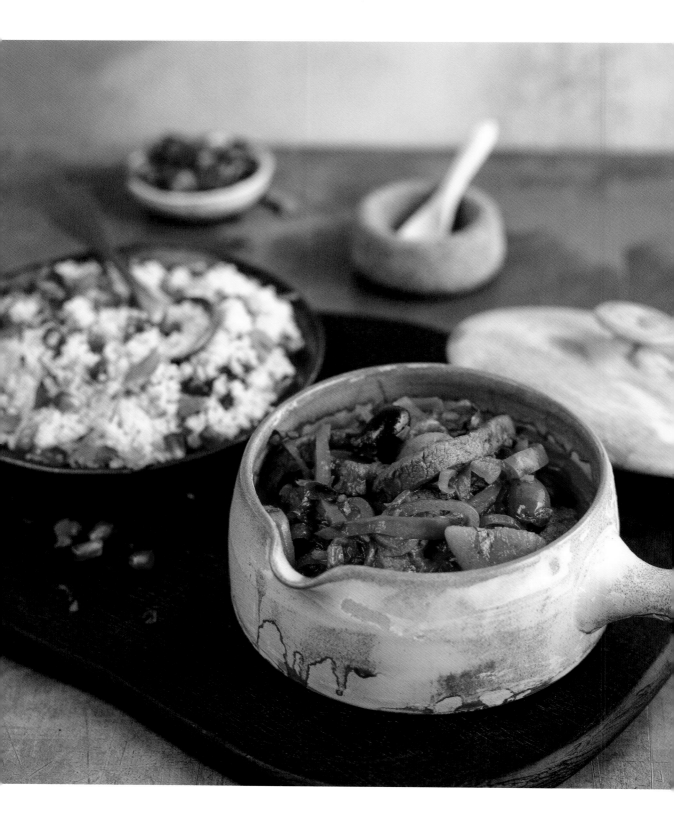

MOROCCAN BEEF
and APRICOT TAGINE

This dish is a real time-saver as it doesn't take a lot of preparation: you just cook the onions and garlic then throw in all the other ingredients, including the beef.

The apricots add a delicious sweetness to the dish that complements all the flavours. If you don't have apricots, then sultanas or raisins would work just as well. If you were a purist, this dish would most likely be made using lamb but as the macronutrients aren't very good (lamb is a rather fatty cut of meat), I've opted for beef instead, which keeps the fat content, and calories, down.

INGREDIENTS

1 tbsp olive or coconut oil
2 red onions, very thinly sliced
1 red pepper, very thinly sliced
2 garlic cloves, crushed
2 tbsp Moroccan spice mix such as
  ras el hanout
500g steak, sliced
2 tbsp tomato purée
10 dried apricots, chopped
10 black pitted olives
500ml vegetable stock

In a large pan, heat the oil over a medium to low heat and add the onion and red pepper. Cook for around 5–10 minutes until cooked through.

Add the garlic and cook for a further minute.

Add the spice mix, steak, tomato purée, apricots, olives and stock to the pan and mix through.

Cover with a lid and then gently simmer for 25–30 minutes until the sauce has thickened.

Serve with couscous.

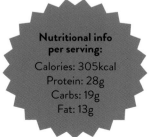

Nutritional info
per serving:
Calories: 305kcal
Protein: 28g
Carbs: 19g
Fat: 13g

Prep time: 10 minutes
Cook time: 30–40 minutes
Serves: 4

ORANGE BEEF

243
CALORIES
per serving

You'll find a version of Orange Beef on lots of Chinese takeaway menus, and for good reason. If you can't find rice wine, or mirin, in your supermarket, you can use the same amount of white wine but add half a teaspoon of sugar for every tablespoon you use, so for this recipe it would be two tablespoons of white wine and one teaspoon sugar. But most supermarkets sell it and I've used it in a few recipes, so hopefully it won't go to waste.

INGREDIENTS

2 tbsp cornflour
½ tsp Chinese 5 spice
Black pepper
500g quick-fry beef, sliced
2 tsp coconut oil
1 red pepper, sliced
1 onion, sliced
1 garlic clove, crushed
1 tsp minced ginger
150ml fresh orange juice (bits or without, it doesn't matter)
150ml chicken stock
½ tsp chilli flakes plus extra for garnish
2 tbsp rice wine
2 tbsp soy sauce
1 orange, sliced, for garnish (optional)
Fresh chives, chopped (optional)
Sesame seeds (optional)

Mix the cornflour, 5 spice seasoning and black pepper in a bowl and add the beef strips. Mix through so it's all coated in the floury mixture.

Heat a wok on a high heat, add 1 teaspoon of coconut oil and fry the beef until cooked through. Remove from the pan and set aside.

Pour in the remaining teaspoon of coconut oil, add the red pepper and onion and fry for a few minutes. Add the garlic and ginger and fry for 30 seconds more.

Pour in the orange juice, stock, chilli flakes, rice wine and soy sauce, put the beef back in the pan and simmer for a few minutes until the sauce has thickened to your desired consistency.

Serve with rice and some sliced orange for garnish along with chopped chives, sesame seeds and chilli flakes.

Nutritional info per serving:
Calories: 243kcal
Protein: 28g
Carbs: 17g
Fat: 7g

Prep time: 10 minutes
Cook time: 15 minutes
Serves: 4

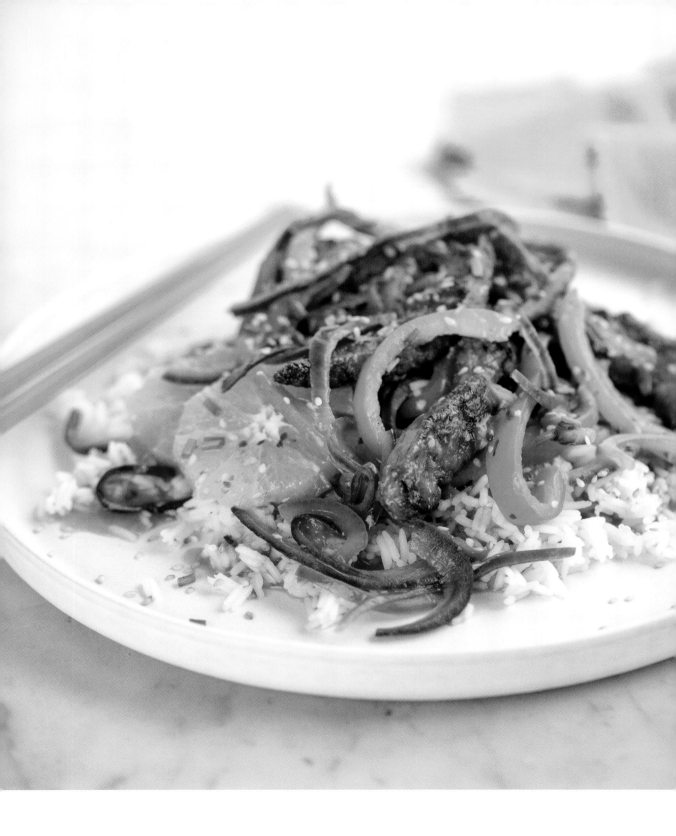

MEXICAN-STYLE LASAGNE

303 CALORIES per serving

If you're looking for a recipe to kick things off, you won't be disappointed with Mexican Lasagne. I'll hold my hands up, I would be pretty amazed if this was actually eaten anywhere in Mexico but I've borrowed inspiration from the fajita and enchilada kits I ate as a student and crossed them with lasagne and here we go. Cheesy, meaty, rich, flavoursome – you can't really go wrong.

INGREDIENTS

1 tbsp coconut or olive oil
3 mixed peppers, chopped
1 green chilli, deseeded and chopped
1 red onion, chopped
2 garlic cloves, chopped
750g 5%-fat beef mince
170g tin sweetcorn, drained
2 x 400g tins chopped tomatoes
3 tbsp fajita or Mexican fajita seasoning
2 tbsp tomato purée
150g low-fat cheddar cheese, grated
4 healthy-living tortilla wraps (the ones that are about 100 calories each)

Preheat the oven to 180°C (160°C fan)/350°F/gas 4. Heat the coconut oil in a large pan and add the pepper, chilli, onion and garlic and cook for a few minutes.

Add mince to the pan and brown it.

Add the sweetcorn, chopped tomatoes, Mexican seasoning and tomato purée to the pan, reduce the heat and simmer for 10–15 minutes.

Once it's cooked, take a large ovenproof lasagne dish and spread a layer of the meat mixture on the bottom, then layer with two of the tortillas (rip them up if necessary). Repeat with another layer of mince and tortillas, then a final layer of mince.

Top with grated cheese and place in the oven for 30 minutes. Serve.

Nutritional info per serving:
Calories: 303kcal
Protein: 30g
Carbs: 21g
Fat: 11g

Prep time: 15 minutes
Cook time: 1 hour
Serves: 8

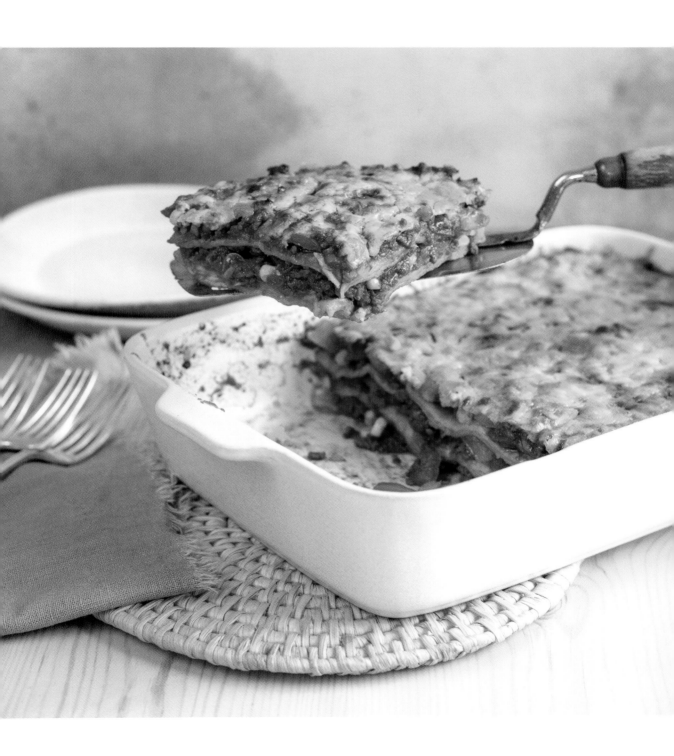

SILKY BEEF

376
CALORIES
per serving

This recipe was originally going to be a beef satay with peanut as one of the dominant flavours. But once I started making it I realised that, although the peanut butter doesn't impart a strong peanutty flavour, it does give the dish a really smooth silky texture, hence satay beef became silky beef. Instead of messing about and trying to make it more satay-esque, and probably jacking up the calories as a result, I decided to include it as it is. This goes well with rice and extra stir-fried vegetables or broccoli.

INGREDIENTS

2 tsp coconut oil
500g frying beef steaks, sliced
1 onion, chopped
150g tinned pineapple (rings or chunks), chopped
1 red pepper, sliced into batons
1 carrot, sliced into batons
2 garlic cloves, crushed
2 tsp minced ginger
½ tsp chilli powder
40g peanut butter
200ml water
1 tbsp soy sauce

Heat a wok on a high heat and add 1 teaspoon of coconut oil. Quickly fry the beef, remove from the pan and set aside.

Pour in the other teaspoon of coconut oil and add the onion, pineapple, pepper and carrot and fry until the vegetables start to darken and the onion turns translucent.

Add the garlic, ginger and chilli powder and fry for a further 30 seconds.

Return the beef to the pan along with the peanut butter, water and soy sauce. Cook for a further few minutes then serve.

Nutritional info per serving:
Calories: 376kcal
Protein 41g
Carbs 17g
Fat 16g

Prep time: 10 minutes
Cook time: 10 minutes
Serves: 3

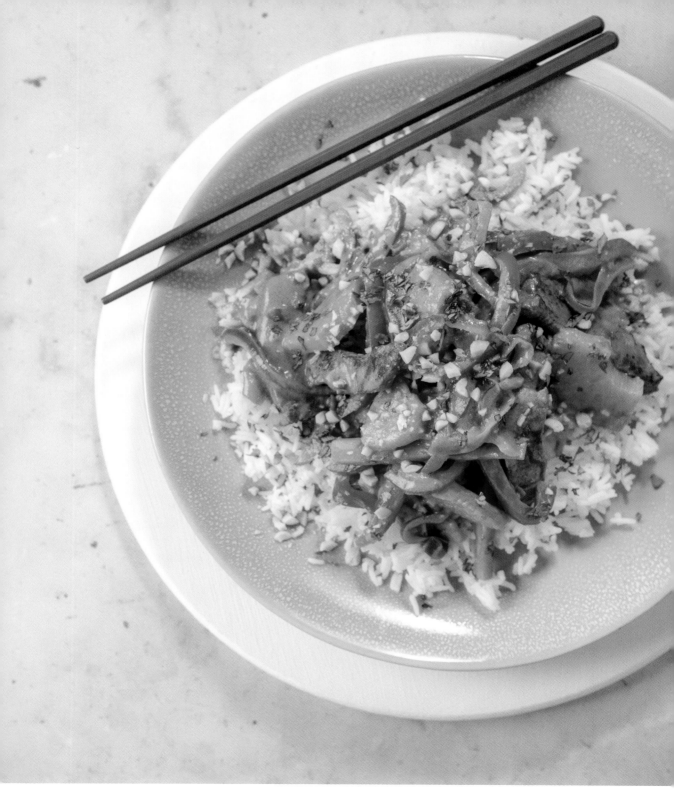

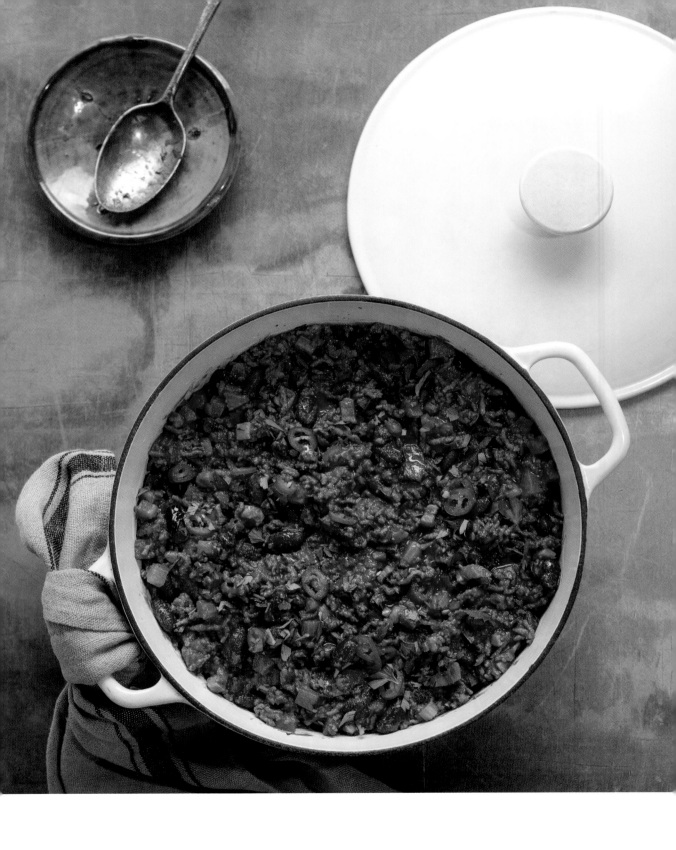

SMOKY BEEF
and BACON CHILLI

360 CALORIES per serving

BEEF

This chilli has officially been dubbed 'the best chilli ever', and not just by me – it's a follower favourite. I think it's the smoked bacon that takes the flavour up a notch. It's also very rich and thick – poles apart from the chilli I remember eating as a kid, which was some mildly spiced mince and kidney beans floating around in tomato juice (sorry mum). As with the Slow-Cooker Peanut Chicken, if you don't have a slow cooker, you can do this in the oven instead. Cook it like a casserole at around 160°C (140°C fan)/315°F/gas 3 for 2–3 hours and double the passata or add 400–500ml of stock.

INGREDIENTS

1 tbsp olive oil
6 smoked bacon medallions, cut into
   small cubes
3 garlic cloves, chopped
1 onion, chopped
800g 5%-fat beef mince
4 stalks celery, chopped
400g tin kidney beans, drained and rinsed
400g passata
2 tbsp tomato purée
1 tbsp chilli powder
1 tbsp ground cumin
1 tbsp smoked paprika
1 tsp salt
2 tbsp Worcestershire sauce

Heat a large frying pan with the olive oil on a medium heat and cook the bacon, garlic and onion for a few minutes until the bacon starts to crisp up, then tip everything into the slow cooker.

Add the mince to the frying pan, increase the heat to high and cook for a few minutes until it's brown, then add it to the slow cooker too.

Add all of the remaining ingredients to the slow cooker, stir, then cover with the lid and cook for 6–8 hours on low.

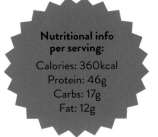

Nutritional info per serving:
Calories: 360kcal
Protein: 46g
Carbs: 17g
Fat: 12g

Prep time: 15 minutes
Cook time: 6–8 hours
Serves: 6

6 335687 751544

TURKISH BEEF STIR-FRY
(SAÇ KAVURMA)

224
CALORIES
per serving

Turkish cuisine is a favourite of mine. I love the spices, the depth of flavour and the fact that every meal I have makes me feel like I am on holiday. Saç kavurma consists of sautéed meat, peppers and spices and takes its name from the traditional metal cooking sheet it's prepared on (not mandatory). Traditionally, it's eaten for breakfast but for me it's a bit heavy for breakfast so I eat it as a main meal. Normally cooked with lamb, I prefer beef, so that's what you get here!

INGREDIENTS

1 tsp olive oil
500g stir-fry beef strips
1 onion, finely chopped
2 peppers, sliced
1 tsp butter
2 tomatoes, chopped
1 tbsp paprika
½ tsp thyme
1 tsp oregano
½ tsp chilli powder
⅓ tsp salt
Fresh parsley, chopped for garnish

Heat a wok or large frying pan on a high heat. Add the olive oil and fry the beef until browned. Remove from the pan and set aside.

Add the onion, sliced pepper and butter and fry until the onion starts to turn golden.

Return the beef to the pan along with the tomato, paprika, herbs, chilli powder and salt, fry for a further 2 minutes then serve.

Garnish with fresh parsley.

**Nutritional info
per serving:**
Calories: 224kcal
Protein: 29g
Carbs: 9g
Fat: 8g

Prep time: 5 minutes
Cook time: 15 minutes
Serves: 4

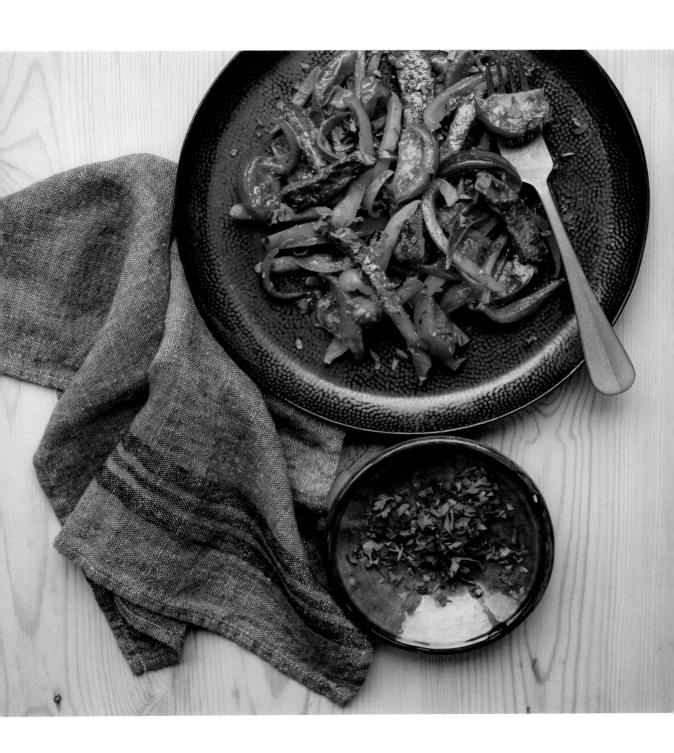

SWEET POTATO STOVIES

360 CALORIES per serving

Stovies is a traditional Scottish dish that is often made on a Monday with leftovers from a weekend roast. It's extremely versatile and you can throw in lots of different ingredients to suit your taste.

I've created a stovies recipe with a twist, using sweet potatoes in place of the traditional white potato (although you can use 'normal' potatoes if you prefer). This recipe also has a couple of other ingredients that you might not find in a normal one, which gives it a really delicious flavour. Some purists might argue that this isn't stovies, but I'd say that it probably tastes better than their version anyway.

This easy recipe takes hardly any time to prepare, it can be scaled up to feed more hungry folks and it can easily be frozen.

INGREDIENTS

700g sweet potatoes, peeled and chopped
1 tsp olive oil
1 red onion, finely diced
1 garlic clove, crushed
500g lean steak mince
4 tsp Worcestershire sauce
30g tomato purée
½ tsp dried rosemary
1 tsp mixed herbs
175ml red wine or stock

Bring a pan of water to the boil and cook the sweet potato pieces for 15–20 minutes until softened.

Meanwhile, heat the olive oil in a large pan over a low to medium heat, add the onion and gently fry for a few minutes. Add the garlic and fry for a further minute before adding the mince to the pan and cooking until it has browned.

Add the Worcestershire sauce, tomato purée, rosemary and mixed herbs with the red wine or stock, cover the pan and simmer for 10 minutes.

Once the sweet potato is ready, drain and mash. Add the mince mixture to the mashed sweet potatoes and thoroughly combine the two.

Serve and enjoy.

Nutritional info per serving:
Calories: 360kcal
Protein: 28g
Carbs: 44g
Fat: 8g

Prep time: 10 minutes
Cook time: 25 minutes
Serves: 4

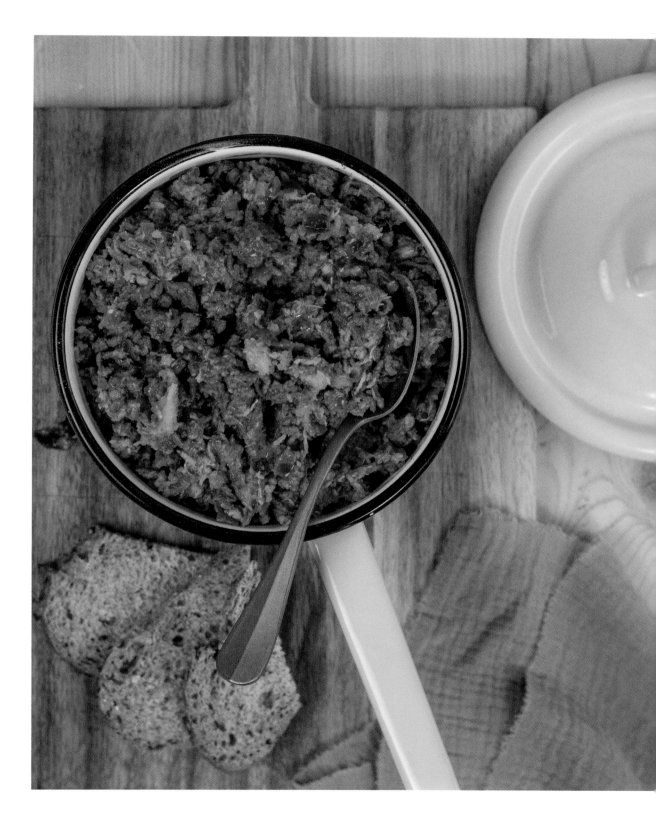

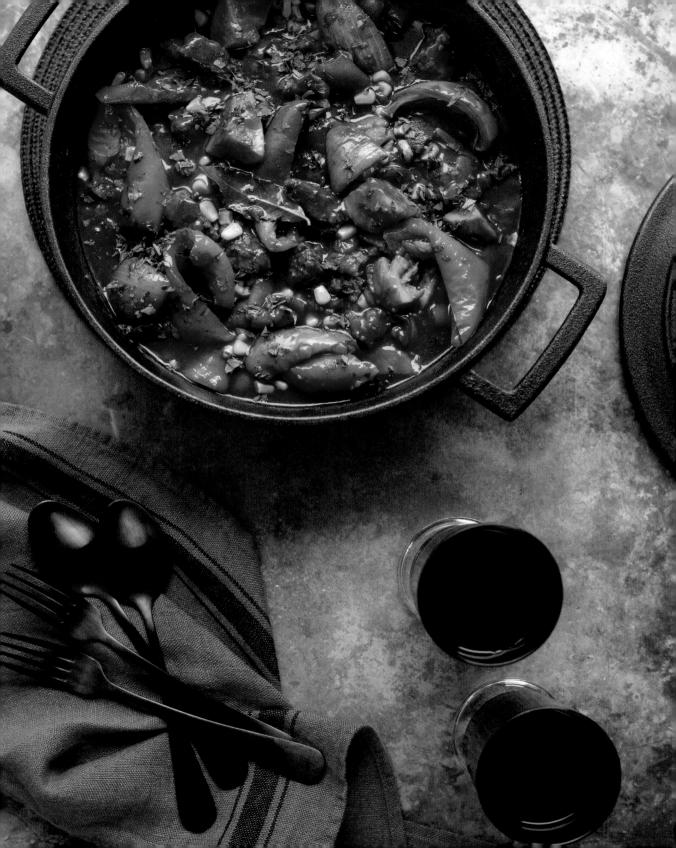

CARBONADA CRIOLLA
(ARGENTINIAN BEEF STEW)

Carbonada Criolla (pronounced *cree-o-sha*) is a beef stew from the Patagonia region of Argentina. At first glance it may look a bit odd, given that you've got a rich, beefy stew with dried apricots and sweetcorn in it but trust me, it's a winning combo. As always, if you want to cut out the booze you can swap the red wine for extra stock. You could also add more sweet potato to bulk out the carbs although you'll need a tad more liquid if you do that. Either way, it's delicious, regardless of how you serve it. *Buen provecho.*

INGREDIENTS

1 tbsp olive oil
1 onion, quartered
1 green pepper, quartered
1 red pepper, quartered
2 garlic cloves, crushed
1kg lean diced beef
400g tin chopped tomatoes
200ml beef stock
200ml red wine
2 sweet potatoes, cut into large chunks
2 bay leaves
1 tbsp paprika
Few grinds of black pepper
150g ready-to-eat dried apricots, sliced
   lengthways
10g cornflour
160g sweetcorn (drained weight)
Fresh parsley, chopped, for garnish

Preheat the oven to 180°C (160°C fan)/350°F/gas 4.

Heat a large ovenproof casserole dish on a medium to high heat, add the olive oil, onion and peppers and fry for a few minutes until the onion starts to brown. Add the garlic and fry for 30 seconds more before adding the beef and browning it for a few minutes.

Add the chopped tomatoes, stock, wine, sweet potato, bay leaves, paprika, pepper, apricots and cornflour and stir through. Bring to the boil, then cover with a lid and place in the oven for 1 hour 30 minutes. Be sure to stir midway through cooking.

When the time is up, add the sweetcorn, stir through and place back in the oven for 10 minutes more.

Remove from the oven and serve garnished with freshly chopped parsley.

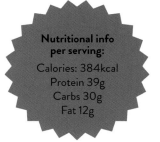

**Nutritional info
per serving:**

Calories: 384kcal
Protein 39g
Carbs 30g
Fat 12g

Prep time: 10 minutes
Cook time: 1 hour 50 minutes
Serves: 6

9 855132 355754

CARBONNADE FLAMANDE

338 CALORIES per serving

Carbonnade Flamande is hands down my favourite beef casserole recipe of all time. Known as *stoofvlees* in the Flemish parts of Belgium, it is delicious, rich and flavoured with beer, bacon, onions and tasty herbs.

When you get this dish in Belgium, it often comes with a plate of frites, but a lower-fat alternative would be pure mashed potatoes. This is also beautiful in a sandwich (we'd call that a 'stew piece' here in Scotland).

INGREDIENTS

1kg lean diced steak
400ml dark beer, eg Leffe Brune or dark IPA
3 garlic cloves, chopped
1 tbsp butter
250g smoked bacon (fat removed), chopped
200g onions, chopped
2 carrots, chopped
40g cornflour
350ml stock
20g tomato purée
2 bay leaves
20g wholegrain mustard
20g honey
1 bouquet garni

Marinate the beef in the beer and garlic for at least 2 hours – the longer the better.

Preheat the oven to 160°C (140°C fan)/315°F/gas 3.

Heat the butter in a large ovenproof dish and fry the bacon, onion and carrot for around 5 minutes or until cooked. Mix in the cornflour.

Add the beef and the liquid marinade along with all the other ingredients.

Mix through, cover and cook in the oven for around 3 hours until tender.

Nutritional info per serving:
Calories: 338kcal
Protein: 46g
Carbs: 16g
Fat: 10g

Prep time: 15 minutes
+ 2 hours to marinate
Cook time: 3 hours 10 minutes
Serves: 6

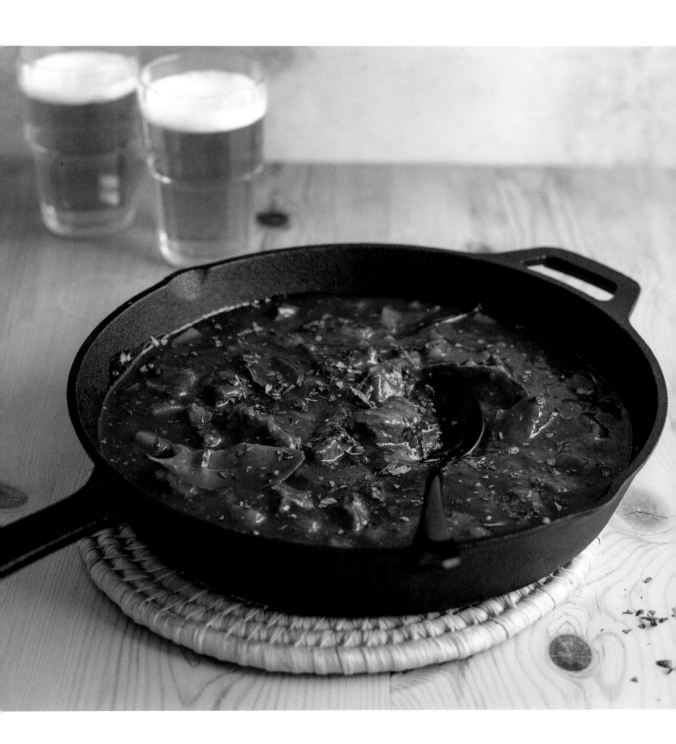

BRAZILIAN COCONUT CHICKEN CURRY

357 CALORIES per serving

This is probably one of the most popular recipes I've ever created or come up with. Arguably you would be hard-pressed to find a Brazilian who used the term 'curry' in the context of their own cuisine. But let me explain: the inspiration for the dish comes from the dish Xim xim, which is enjoyed throughout Brazil and often has crayfish tails in it. Since crayfish are quite hard to find here and not everyone's cup of tea, I tweaked a few Xim xim recipes to come up with this one, which hits the spot and is closer to the kind of curry we're familiar with.

INGREDIENTS

600g chicken breasts, chopped
1 tbsp coconut oil
1 red onion, diced
1 garlic clove, chopped
1 green chilli, deseeded and chopped, plus
  extra for garnish
1 chicken stock cube
Zest and juice of 1 lime
400ml light coconut milk
100ml water
1 tsp ground turmeric
100g peanut butter (crunchy or smooth)
Pinch of black pepper
Fresh coriander, chopped, for garnish

Preheat the oven to 180°C (160°C fan)/350°F/gas 4.

Gently fry the chicken pieces in the coconut oil in a casserole dish or ovenproof saucepan until they are lightly browned, then remove from the pan and set aside.

Add the onion, garlic and chilli to the pan and fry for a minute before crumbling in the stock cube.

Add the lime zest and juice, coconut milk, water, turmeric and peanut butter to the dish and mix through.

Return the chicken to the dish, cover and place in the oven for 35 minutes.

Serve with rice and garnish with chilli slices and fresh coriander.

Nutritional info per serving:
Calories: 357kcal
Protein: 35g
Carbs: 7g
Fat: 21g

Prep time: 10 minutes
Cook time: 50 minutes
Serves: 5

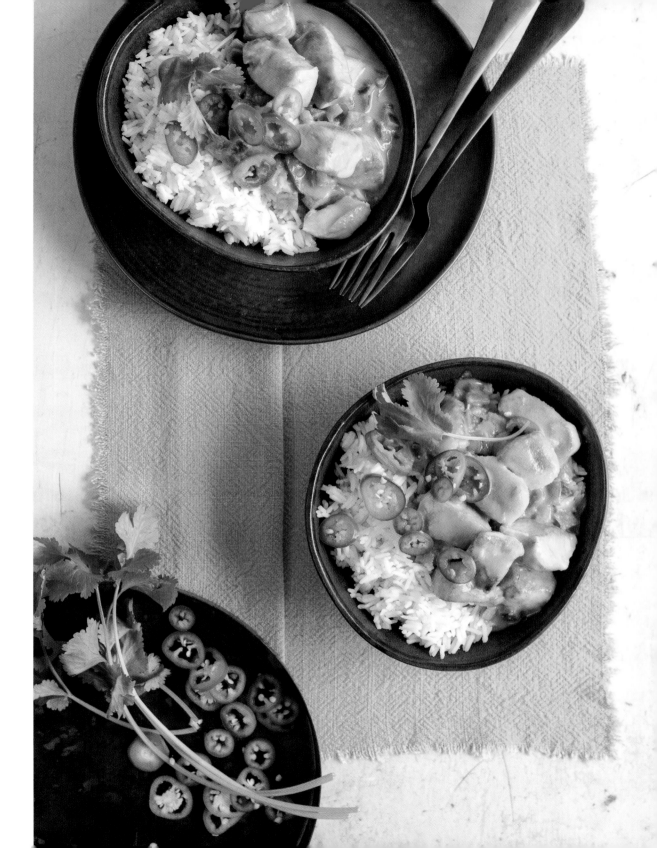

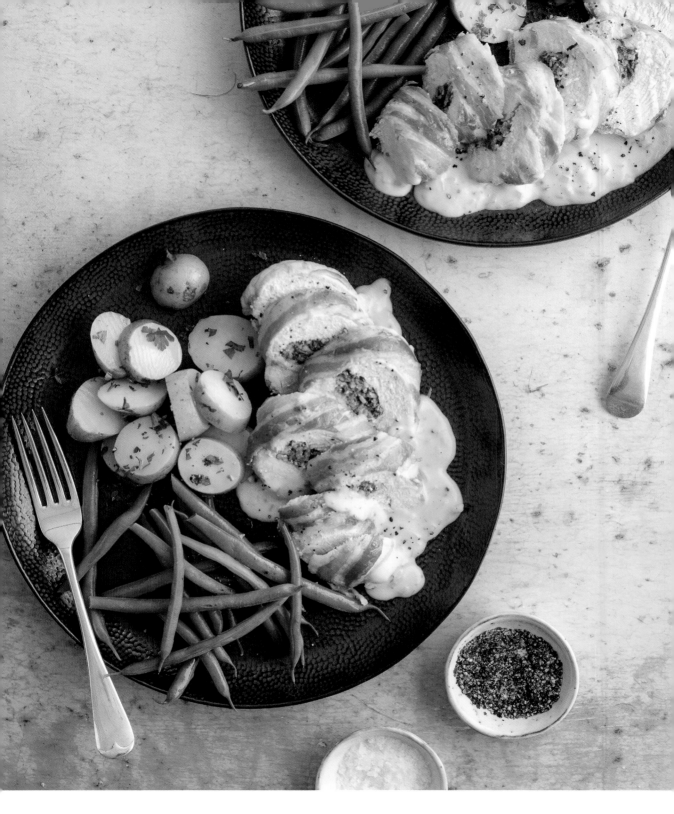

CHICKEN BALMORAL

This is a classic found on pub menus all across Scotland. With two of our most popular exports (haggis and whisky) in the mix, it is the epitome of Scottish cuisine. All it needs is a battered Mars bar on the side and an Irn-Bru to wash it down (please don't do this). This wouldn't normally be classed as a calorie-friendly meal due to the lashings of double cream, but I've come up with a much lighter version that still tastes delicious without packing the same calorific punch. Goes brilliantly with potatoes.

INGREDIENTS

500g chicken breasts
150g haggis or black pudding
4 rashers bacon
2 tsp olive oil
1 red onion, finely chopped
50ml whisky
1 tbsp plain flour
400ml chicken stock
1 tsp wholegrain mustard
25ml double cream
Salt and pepper

Preheat the oven to 180°C (160°C fan)/350°F/gas 4.

Slice a pocket into each chicken breast and stuff with some black pudding or haggis. Wrap each breast in a rasher of bacon and use a cocktail stick or butcher's twine to secure it so it doesn't fall apart.

Heat a frying pan on a high heat with 1 teaspoon of olive oil and sear both sides of each chicken breast, then transfer to a baking dish and bake for 35–40 minutes.

While the chicken is cooking, make the sauce. Heat a small pan on a medium heat. Add the remaining 1 teaspoon of oil and the onion and fry until it's turning translucent.

Pour in the whisky and reduce until it has almost completely evaporated. Add the plain flour and mix through. Add the stock, mustard and black pepper. Pour the contents of the pan into a blender and blitz until smooth.

Return the sauce to the pan and simmer until it reaches your desired thickness. Just before serving with the chicken, stir through the cream and season to taste.

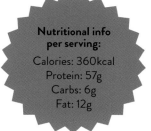
Nutritional info per serving:
Calories: 360kcal
Protein: 57g
Carbs: 6g
Fat: 12g

1 462234 043823

Prep time: 15 minutes
Cook time: 40 minutes
Serves: 4

CHICKEN PILAU

482
CALORIES
per serving

Some followers may know this one as 'Chicken Biryani' but for the sake of accuracy a biryani is made with layers of rice and meat, whereas this recipe is closer to a pilau. Anyway, this is a popular one-pot recipe that can be thrown in the oven and largely forgotten about until it's ready. It's a winner of a dish, even though there is a debate about whether it should or shouldn't have raisins in it. Personally, I love the sweetness they add. Unlike most recipes in this book, I don't think this one keeps or reheats well so you're best eating it fresh, which is no hardship as it's very moreish.

INGREDIENTS

1 tbsp coconut oil
500g chicken breasts, chopped
1 garlic clove, crushed
1 tsp ground turmeric
½ tsp chilli powder
1 large onion, finely chopped
2 tbsp curry powder
200g basmati rice
80g raisins
200g frozen peas
750ml chicken stock

Preheat the oven to 180°C (160°C fan)/350°F/gas 4.

In a large ovenproof pan heat the coconut oil and gently fry the chicken on a low heat. Cook until golden brown and thoroughly cooked through (around 10 minutes).

Add the garlic, turmeric, chilli powder and chopped onion to the pan and cook until the onion starts to turn translucent. Add the curry powder, uncooked rice, raisins, peas and stock, cover and bring to the boil.

Once it starts to boil, place the pan in the oven and bake for 35 minutes until all the liquid has been absorbed.

**Nutritional info
per serving:**
Calories: 482kcal
Protein: 39g
Carbs: 68g
Fat: 6g

Prep time: 10 minutes
Cook time: 55 minutes
Serves: 4

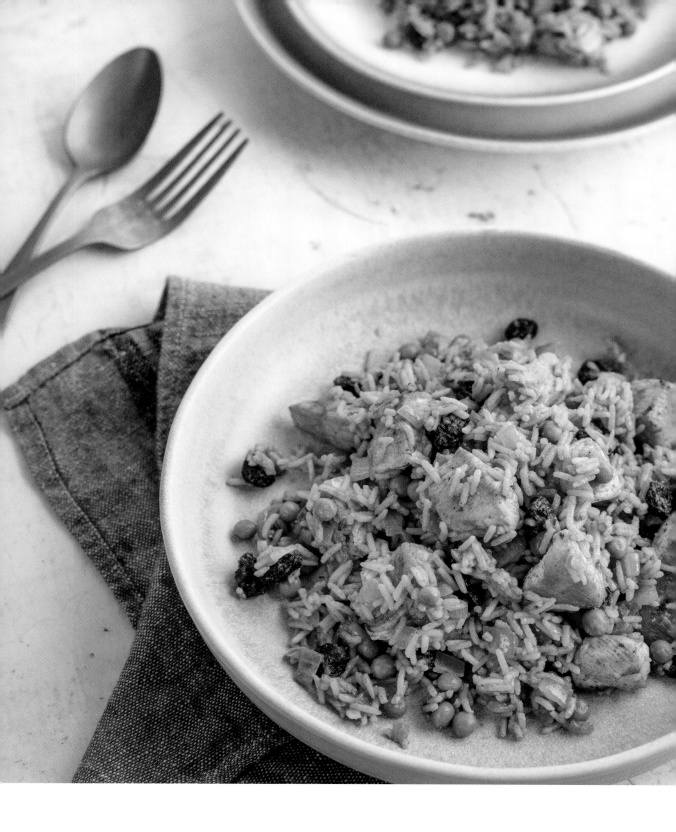

CREAMY WHITE WINE CHICKEN

359 CALORIES per serving

The booze, mushrooms, shallots and garlic give this recipe a real hit of flavour, but the crème fraîche gives it a delicious creaminess that takes it to the next level. If you've not got any shallots, onions, preferably red, work fine. Turkey steaks are also really good in this recipe. For sides, I think it works well with rice and any vegetables.

INGREDIENTS

1 tbsp olive oil
500g chicken breasts, sliced down the middle into steaks
Few grinds of black pepper
3 shallots, finely chopped
1 garlic clove, finely chopped
80g mushrooms, sliced
150ml white wine
150ml chicken stock
1 tsp mixed herbs
100ml reduced-fat crème fraîche
Fresh parsley, chopped, for garnish

Heat the olive oil in a frying pan on a medium to high heat. Season the chicken breasts with black pepper then pan fry for 3–5 minutes per side until they start to turn golden brown. They don't need to be fully cooked through at this stage, just about 80 per cent there.

Once ready, remove from the pan and set aside. Add the shallot, garlic and mushrooms and fry for a further couple of minutes until the onion starts to turn translucent.

Return the chicken to the pan along with the white wine. Allow the wine to reduce to almost nothing then add the stock, mixed herbs and crème fraîche.

Reduce the heat to a simmer and cook for 5 more minutes or until the sauce has thickened and the chicken is fully cooked through.

Serve in the frying pan with fresh parsley for garnish.

Nutritional info per serving:
Calories: 359kcal
Protein: 52g
Carbs: 4g
Fat: 15g

Prep time: 10 minutes
Cook time: 15–20 minutes
Serves: 3

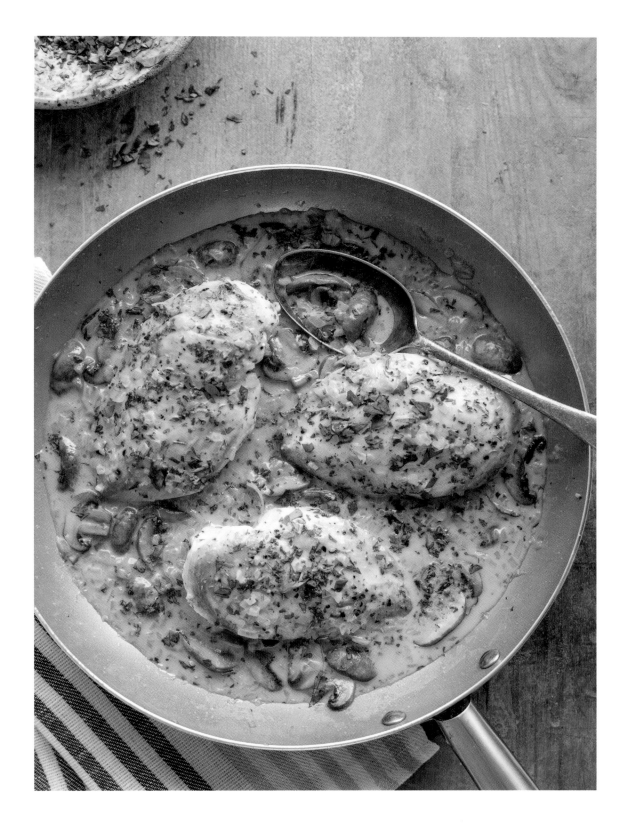

ST MARY'S CHICKEN

316 CALORIES per serving

I did my Sports Nutrition Masters at St Mary's University, Twickenham. One of the classes was recipe preparation for athletes and one day we were given a handful of ingredients and told to come up with a recipe. Kind of like *Ready Steady Cook* if you remember that? Anyway, this is what I came up with and it's proved hugely popular, even with people who say they don't like mustard.

INGREDIENTS

500g chicken breasts, chopped
6 rashers bacon (fat removed) or bacon medallions, chopped
1 garlic clove, crushed
200ml chicken stock
10g wholegrain mustard
100ml full-fat crème fraîche
1 tsp dried thyme
10g cornflour
30g honey
Pinch of black pepper

Preheat the oven to 180°C (160°C fan)/350°F/gas 4.

Arrange the chicken breasts in an ovenproof dish and sprinkle them with the chopped bacon.

In a jug, mix the garlic, stock, mustard, crème fraîche, thyme, cornflour, honey and pepper. Pour the mixture over the chicken.

Bake in the oven for 40-45 minutes until the chicken is thoroughly cooked through. Serve with green veg, new potatoes or rice.

Nutritional info per serving:
Calories: 316kcal
Protein: 41g
Carbs: 11g
Fat: 12g

Prep time: 10 minutes
Cook time: 45 minutes
Serves: 4

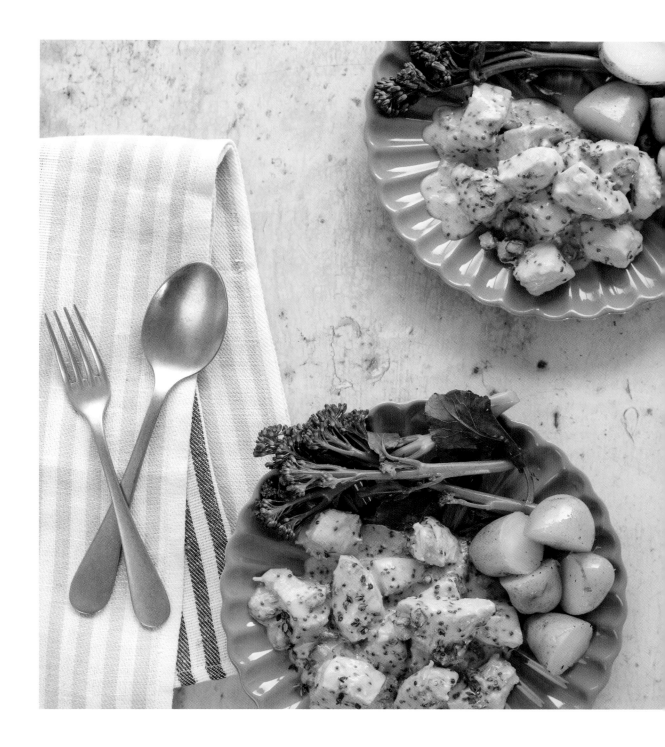

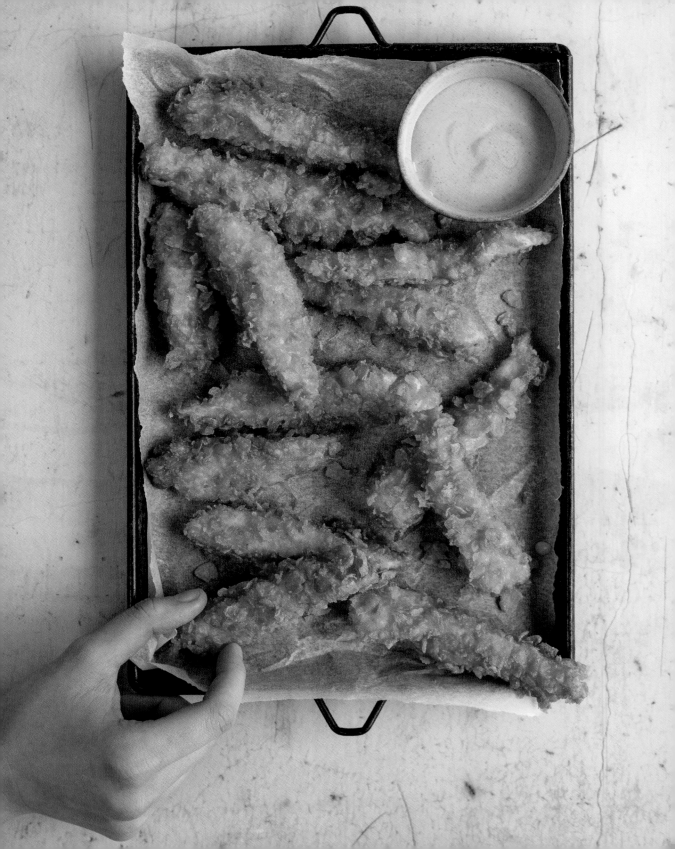

CRISPY CORNFLAKE CHICKEN

336
CALORIES
per serving

This is my take on a KFC so if you're a fan of fakeaway recipes, you should enjoy this leaner, healthier alternative. The spice mix at KFC is one of food's most closely-guarded secrets, but I think we're pretty much there with this combo. Great eaten straight away for maximum crunch and crispiness but can be reheated. If you like a bit of heat with your chicken, add some chilli powder in the seasoning.

INGREDIENTS

80g cornflakes
2 tbsp plain flour
1 tsp mixed herbs
1 tsp salt
2 tsp paprika
1 tsp garlic powder
Pinch of ginger powder
500g chicken, cut into fillets
1 egg, whisked

Preheat the oven to 180°C (160°C fan)/350°F/gas 4.

Crush the cornflakes in a bowl. Mix the flour with the herbs and all the seasoning.

Coat the chicken pieces in the flour, dip them in the egg then dip the pieces into the cornflakes. Place the chicken on a baking tray lined with greaseproof paper.

Cook for 10–15 minutes, turn the chicken, then cook for a further 10–15 minutes until thoroughly cooked through. Serve.

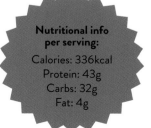

Nutritional info
per serving:
Calories: 336kcal
Protein: 43g
Carbs: 32g
Fat: 4g

Prep time: 15 minutes
Cook time: 20–30 minutes
Serves: 3

7 071398 543540

CREAMY CAJUN CHICKEN PASTA

555 CALORIES per serving

This is another great one for midweek and should be a crowd-pleaser. You pretty much make fajitas but use pasta instead of a wrap and mix through some crème fraîche. What's not to like? Use more or less fajita seasoning (Cajun spice mix also works well) depending on how hot you like it and feel free to bung in other veg too. I've cooked this with courgette, carrots and green beans, etc.

INGREDIENTS

300g pasta (dry weight)
2 tsp olive oil
400g chicken breasts, chopped
3 bacon medallions, chopped
1 onion, chopped
1 red pepper, chopped
1 green pepper, chopped
160g sweetcorn (drained weight)
2 tsp fajita seasoning
100ml half-fat crème fraîche
½ bunch of fresh coriander, chopped
Lime wedges

Cook the pasta following the instructions on the packet.

Heat 1 teaspoon of olive oil in a pan on a medium to high heat and fry the chicken pieces until golden. Once cooked, remove from the pan and set aside.

Add the second teaspoon of oil to the pan along with the bacon, onion, peppers and corn and fry until the corn starts to brown.

Return the chicken to the pan with the fajita seasoning and cook for a further minute.

Drain the pasta (keeping some water) and add to the chicken and vegetables with the crème fraîche and a little pasta water, if needed, to loosen everything up.

Serve with coriander and lime wedges.

Nutritional info per serving:
Calories: 555kcal
Protein: 48g
Carbs: 66g
Fat: 11g

Prep time: 10 minutes
Cook time: 25 minutes
Serves: 4

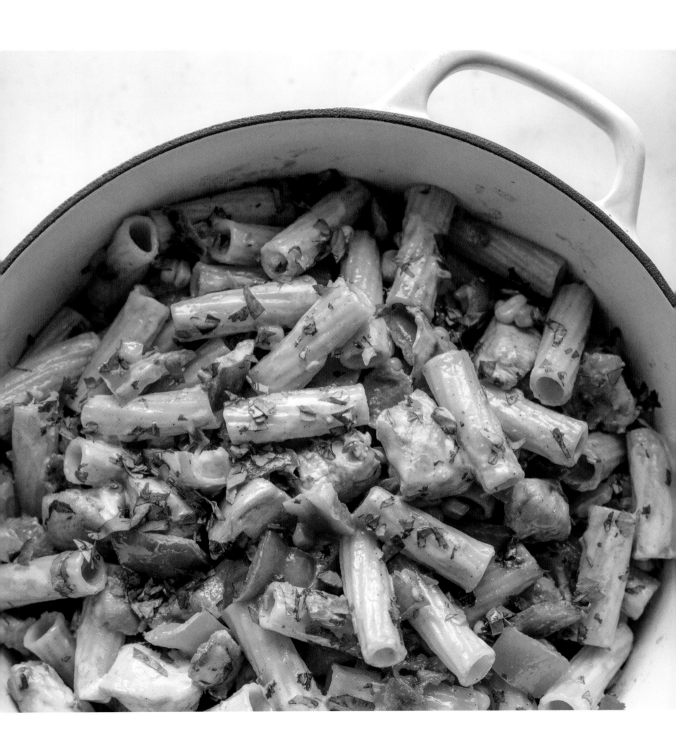

PEANUT CHICKEN

329
CALORIES
per serving

This is like a satay but not so nutty and more tomato-y. As you'll see, the method has just two steps so that on its own makes this a winner, especially if you're looking for a midweek time saver. This recipe can easily be scaled up if your slow cooker is big enough. If you don't have a slow cooker, fear not. You can cook it like a casserole in the oven, at 160°C (140°C fan)/315°F/gas 3 for a few hours, doubling the chopped tomatoes or adding about 500ml of stock. Enjoy!

INGREDIENTS

1kg chicken breasts, diced
1 onion, chopped
2 garlic cloves, crushed
120g peanut butter (crunchy or smooth)
1 tbsp cornflour
400g tin chopped tomatoes
1 red chilli, deseeded
2 tbsp lime juice
1 tbsp curry powder
2 tbsp soy sauce

Throw all of the ingredients into the slow cooker.

Cover and cook on low for 5 hours.

Nutritional info per serving:
Calories: 329kcal
Protein: 43g
Carbs: 10g
Fat: 13g

Prep time: 10 minutes
Cook time: 5 hours
Serves: 6

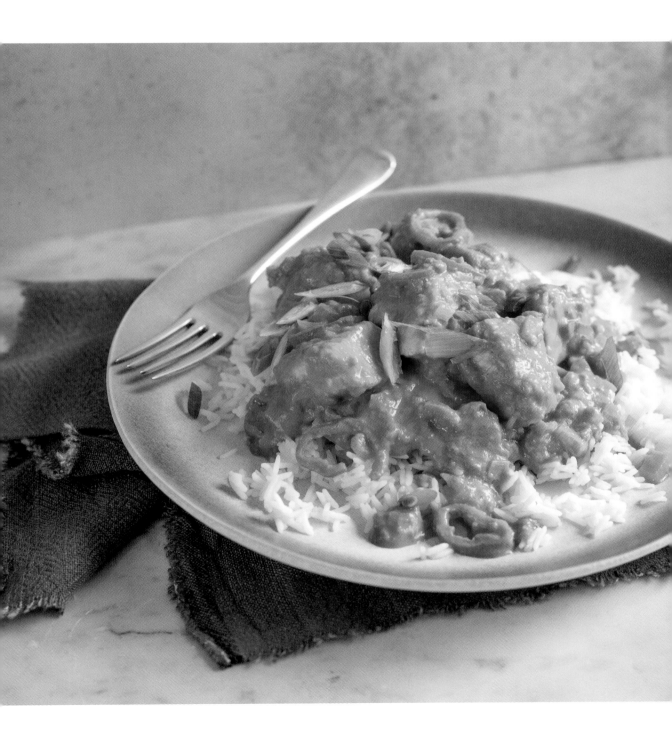

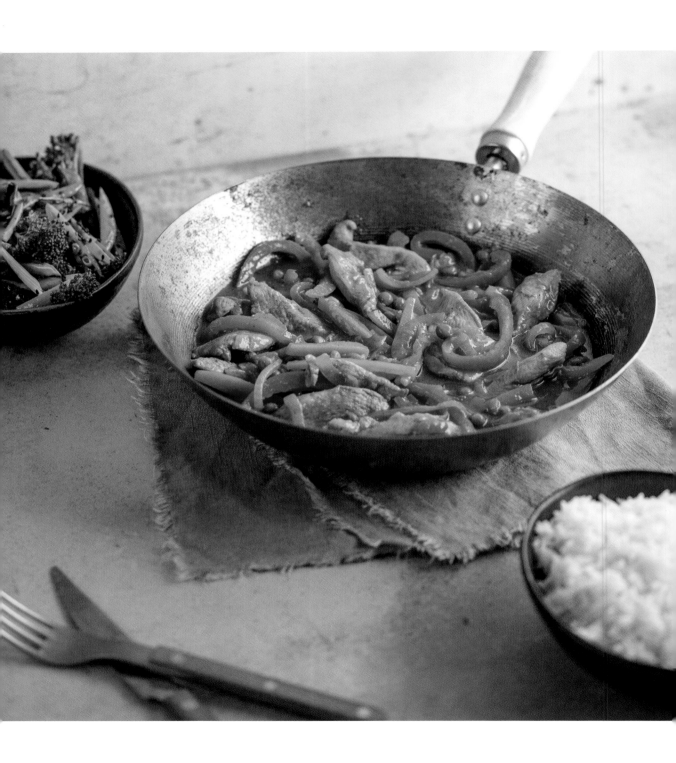

CHINESE TAKEAWAY CHICKEN CURRY

325
CALORIES
per serving

If you're partial to a curry from your local Chinese, then this recipe is going to save you a few quid! Not only that, but I think you'll be hard-pressed to tell the difference – this one is pretty authentic. It's a doozie, very quick to make and should be a crowd-pleaser if you do a #FakeawayFriday. Use beef, pork or prawns for the protein source if you want to mix things up. Goes really well with rice (boiled or fried) and stir-fried vegetables.

INGREDIENTS

1 tbsp coconut oil
2 onions, sliced
1 red pepper, sliced
1 carrot, sliced into batons
2 garlic cloves, crushed
2 tsp minced ginger
10g curry powder
20g cornflour
500ml chicken stock
40ml light soy sauce
10g honey
500g chicken breasts, finely sliced
50g frozen peas

Heat the coconut oil in a wok on a high heat. Add the onion, pepper and carrot and fry until they're turning golden. Add the garlic and ginger and fry for 1 minute more. Sprinkle in the curry powder and cornflour and mix through.

Pour in the stock, soy sauce, honey, add the chicken slices and combine. Reduce the heat to a simmer and cook for around 20 minutes. A few minutes before the end of the cooking time, add the peas and cook for a further 3–4 minutes until they're heated through.

Serve.

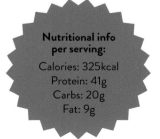

Nutritional info
per serving:

Calories: 325kcal
Protein: 41g
Carbs: 20g
Fat: 9g

Prep time: 15 minutes
Cook time: 30 minutes
Serves: 4

7 502659 301772

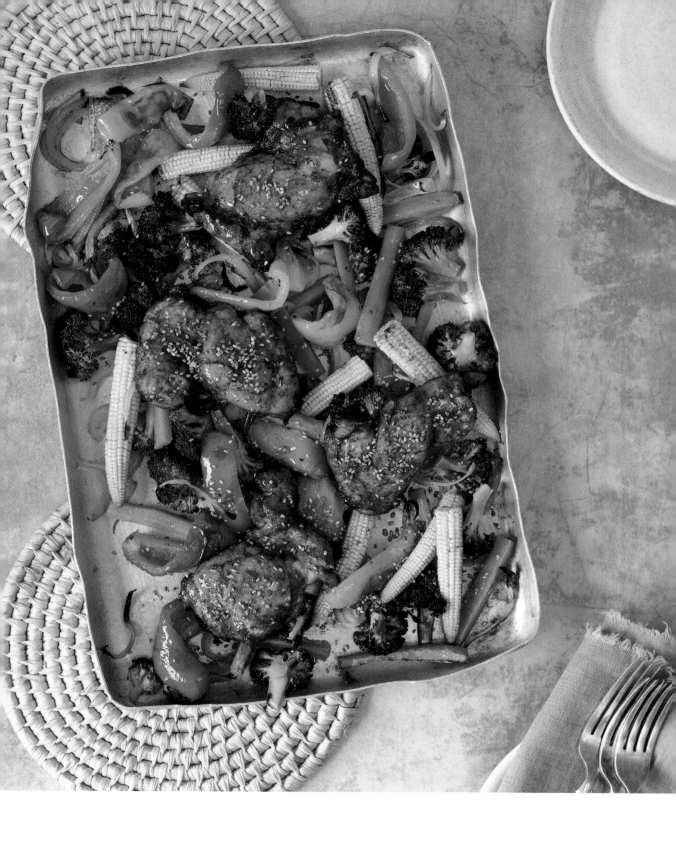

CHINESE CHICKEN TRAYBAKE

Traybakes are a midweek meal staple. Bung everything onto a tray, veg and all, throw it into the oven and Bob's your father's brother. We're going for chicken thighs in this recipe as they retain moisture a lot better than chicken breasts in the oven, but you could swap for chicken breasts to reduce the calories. As always, marinating for longer will give you more flavour and feel free to throw any other vegetables into the mix too.

INGREDIENTS

1 tbsp reduced-salt soy sauce
50ml oyster sauce
1 tbsp rice wine vinegar
1 tsp five-spice powder
2 garlic cloves, crushed
2 tsp minced ginger
500g chicken thigh fillets, chopped
½ head of broccoli, chopped into florets
1 red pepper, sliced
1 yellow pepper, sliced
1 onion, sliced
1 large carrot, sliced into batons
Handful of baby corn
1 tbsp sesame oil

Combine the soy sauce, oyster sauce, rice wine vinegar, five spice, garlic and ginger in a bowl and add the chicken thigh fillets. Place into the fridge to marinate for at least an hour, the longer the better.

Once ready, preheat the oven to 200°C (180°C fan)/400°F/gas 6.

Tip the vegetables onto a baking tray and add the sesame oil. Mix through so the vegetables are all coated. Place into the oven and bake for 10 minutes.

Remove from the oven and place the chicken on top of the vegetables. Pour the leftover marinade over the top.

Return to the oven and bake for about 20 minutes more, ensuring the chicken is thoroughly cooked through before serving.

Prep time: 10 mins + 1 hour to marinate
Cook time: 30 minutes
Serves: 3

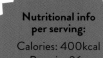

Nutritional info
per serving:
Calories: 400kcal
Protein: 36g
Carbs: 19g
Fat: 20g

PERI-PERI CHICKEN

447
CALORIES
per serving

Bring the flavours of Portugal to your dinner table with this dish, which is perfect for barbecuing. The slaw is a yummy side that will work well with a lot of other recipes too. As always, you can swap things around and I've cooked this with chicken thighs before, which was great but obviously higher in calories. If you like your chicken hot and spicy, just add a touch more peri-peri. Conversely, if you've got quite sensitive taste buds you might find a full teaspoon is too much.

INGREDIENTS

Chicken

1kg chicken breasts
1 tbsp olive oil
Juice of 1 lemon (about 30ml)
1 tsp Worcestershire sauce
2 tsp soy sauce
1 tsp peri-peri seasoning

Coleslaw

½ head of cabbage, finely sliced
1 carrot, grated
1 red onion, finely sliced
1 tbsp apple cider vinegar
100g light mayonnaise
100g low-fat Greek yoghurt

2 corn on the cobs, halved

Mix all the chicken ingredients together and leave to marinate for at least 30 minutes.

Mix all the coleslaw ingredients together.

Cook the chicken on a barbecue, griddle pan or under a grill with the halved corn cobs.

Serve the chicken with a dollop of coleslaw and the corn on the cob.

**Nutritional info
per serving:**
Calories: 447kcal
Protein: 65g
Carbs: 13g
Fat: 15g

Prep time: 15 minutes +
30 minutes to marinate
Cook time: 15 minutes
Serves: 5

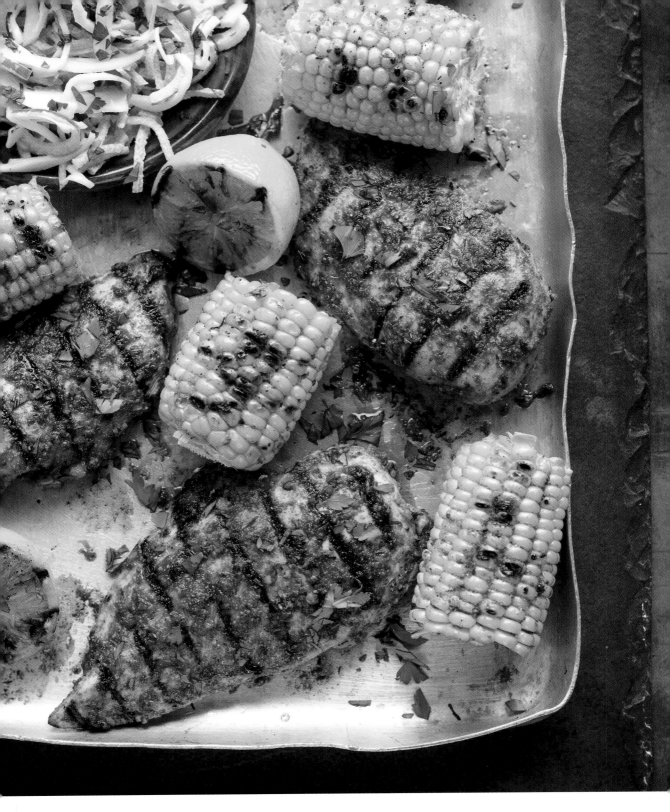

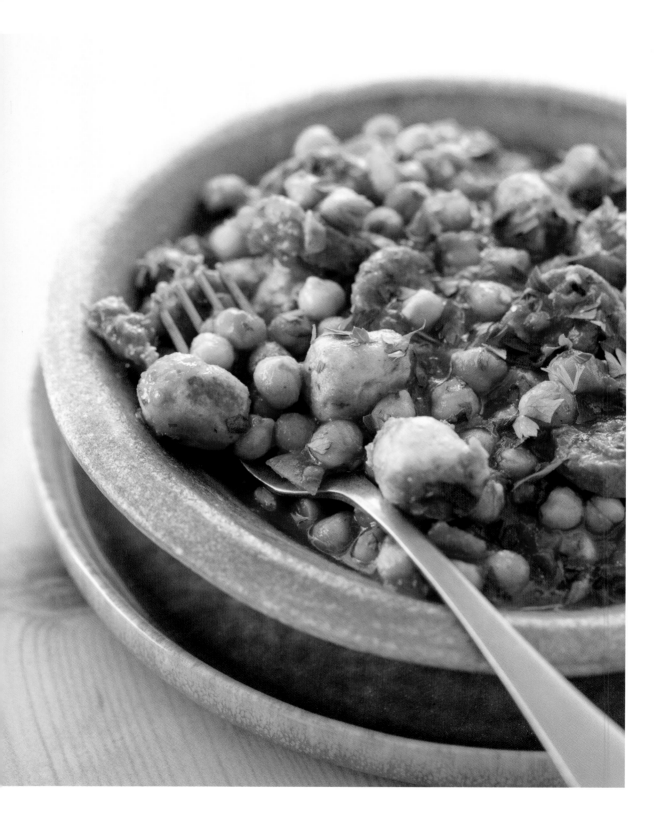

CHORIZO, CHICKEN *and* CHICKPEA STEW

304 CALORIES per serving

I came up with this after I got some delicious chorizo in a Spanish food hamper for my birthday. It's a rich, warming, Mediterranean stew packed with protein from the sausages and chickpeas, with smoked paprika and chorizo adding delicious Spanish-style flavours. You can serve it as is in a bowl or dunk some crusty bread into it. It goes well with rice and potatoes too. Truth be told, it's probably one of my favourites in this book. Hopefully you'll agree!

INGREDIENTS

100g chorizo, sliced
300g low-fat chicken sausages, chopped
1 red onion, finely chopped
2 garlic cloves, finely chopped
½ tsp cumin seeds
1 tsp oregano
1 tsp smoked paprika
400g tin chopped tomatoes
400g can chickpeas, drained and rinsed
300-600ml chicken stock
2 tbsp tomato purée

Heat a large pan on a medium heat and gently fry the chorizo, chicken sausage pieces and red onion for about 10 minutes. You probably won't need to add oil as enough should be released from the chorizo (if you do, add a tiny bit of olive oil).

Add the garlic and cumin seeds and fry for a further minute.

Add the oregano, smoked paprika, chopped tomatoes, chickpeas and tomato purée. Add 300ml stock to begin with and simmer for 15-20 minutes, uncovered, until the sauce has thickened. Add more stock if the sauce it too thick. Serve.

Prep time: 10 minutes
Cook time: 35 minutes
Serves: 4

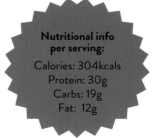

Nutritional info
per serving:
Calories: 304kcals
Protein: 30g
Carbs: 19g
Fat: 12g

3 663450 528691

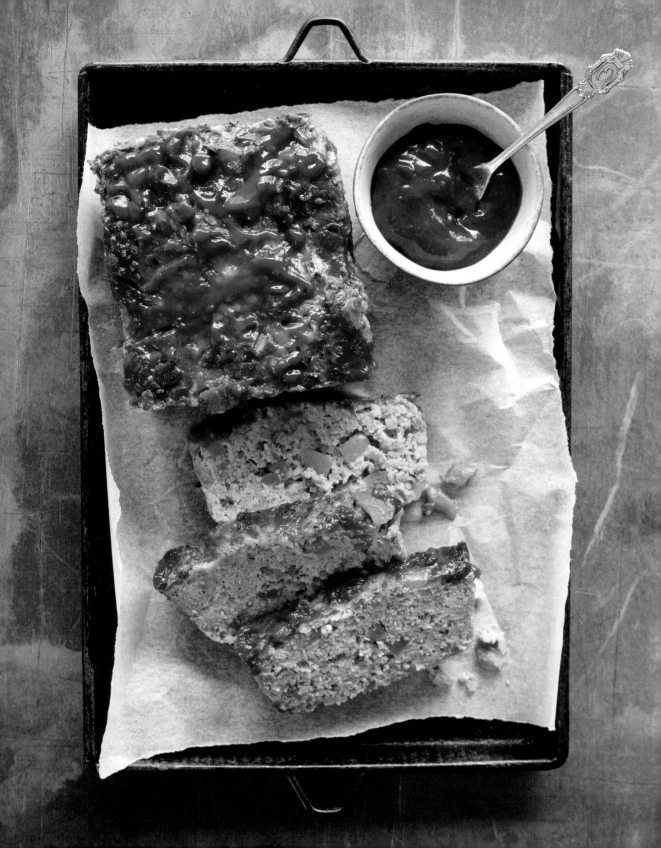

AMERICAN-STYLE BBQ MEATLOAF

This easy meatloaf recipe takes only a few minutes to prepare and tastes pretty authentically American. The meat is juicy and packed with flavour and the BBQ sauce gives it a beautiful sweet topping. You can also make a delicious gravy using the juices: once the meatloaf is cooked, just pour the cooking juices into a pan and add some gravy granules to make a rich sauce to douse it.

INGREDIENTS

500g 5%-fat pork mince
1 onion, grated
1 pepper (red or green), finely chopped
2 garlic cloves, crushed
50ml milk
2 tbsp BBQ seasoning
25g oats
1 egg
2 tbsp tomato ketchup
2 tbsp BBQ sauce
Butter, for greasing

Preheat the oven to 180°C (160°C fan)/350°F/gas 4.

Mix all the ingredients (except the tomato ketchup, BBQ sauce and butter) in a bowl and use your hands to get it all thoroughly combined.

Grease a loaf tin (600g is standard) with some butter and empty the mixture into it.

Top the meatloaf with the ketchup and BBQ sauce then bake for around 45 minutes.

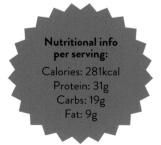

Nutritional info per serving:
Calories: 281kcal
Protein: 31g
Carbs: 19g
Fat: 9g

Prep time: 10 minutes
Cook time: 45 minutes
Serves: 4

4 832376 965456

HONEY *and* ROSEMARY PORK *with* RISOTTO

605 CALORIES per serving

A pork fillet is one of the most underrated cuts of meat there is. It's generally cheaper than chicken or beef, it's very lean, it's versatile and it can be used to make some delicious recipes. When you roast it, as in this recipe, it's so easy to create a tasty meal. This risotto recipe pairs with the pork very well but it's also a great standalone that you could cook (or serve) as a side dish for a lot of other recipes in this book.

INGREDIENTS

Pork
2 tbsp honey
1 tsp Worcestershire sauce
1 tbsp balsamic vinegar
1 garlic clove
1 tsp fresh rosemary
1 tsp olive oil
Few grinds of black pepper
500g pork fillet

Risotto
1 tsp olive oil
1 tsp fennel seeds
½ tsp chopped fresh rosemary
1 onion, finely chopped
1 garlic clove, crushed
300g arborio rice
150ml white wine
1.5 litres hot chicken stock
50g low-fat cheddar cheese, finely grated
½ small bunch of fresh flat-leaf parsley, finely chopped

Preheat the oven to 180°C (160°C fan)/350°F/gas 4. Mix all the marinade ingredients for the pork in a bowl.

Brown the meat in a frying pan, put it on a baking tray, coat with the marinade and stick in the oven for 15 minutes.

The pork will be cooked before the risotto is ready so be ready to remove it from the oven and leave it in a warm place to rest before slicing it to serve. Meanwhile for the risotto, heat the olive oil in a large pan, add the fennel seeds and rosemary and fry for 30 seconds to infuse the oil with flavour. Add the onion and fry until golden. Add the garlic and fry for a further 30 seconds. Add the rice and coat with the mixture. Pour in the wine and simmer for a few minutes until it's pretty much all absorbed or has evaporated.

Add a ladle of stock and stir until mostly absorbed, then add another ladle and do the same. Keep doing this until the rice is cooked, which will take 18–20 minutes. If you've used all the stock and the rice is still too firm, use boiling water until it's tender.

Remove from the heat, mix through the cheddar and garnish with parsley. Serve with slices of the pork.

Nutritional info per serving:
Calories: 605kcal
Protein: 39g
Carbs: 74g
Fat: 17g

Prep time: 10 minutes
Cook time: 30 minutes
Serves: 4

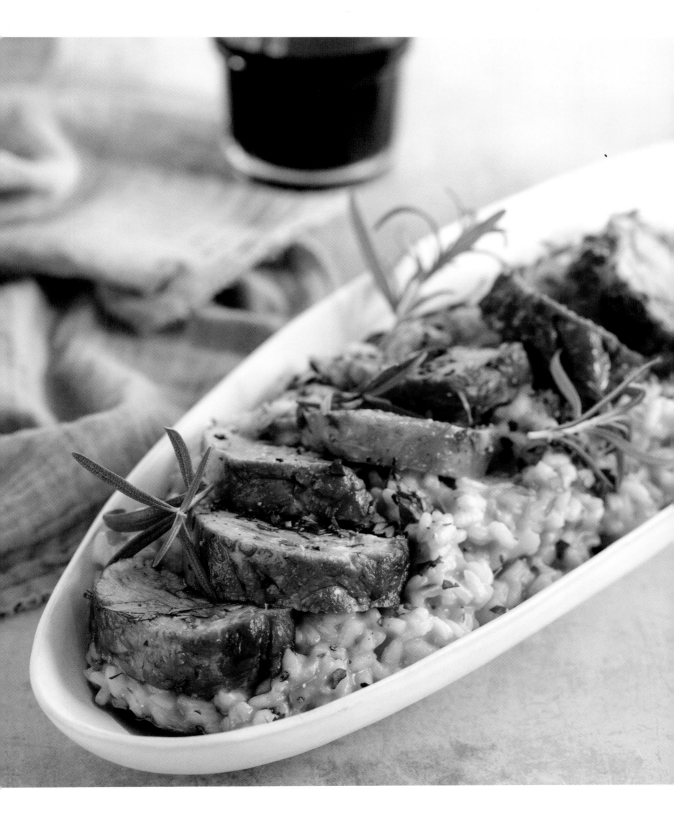

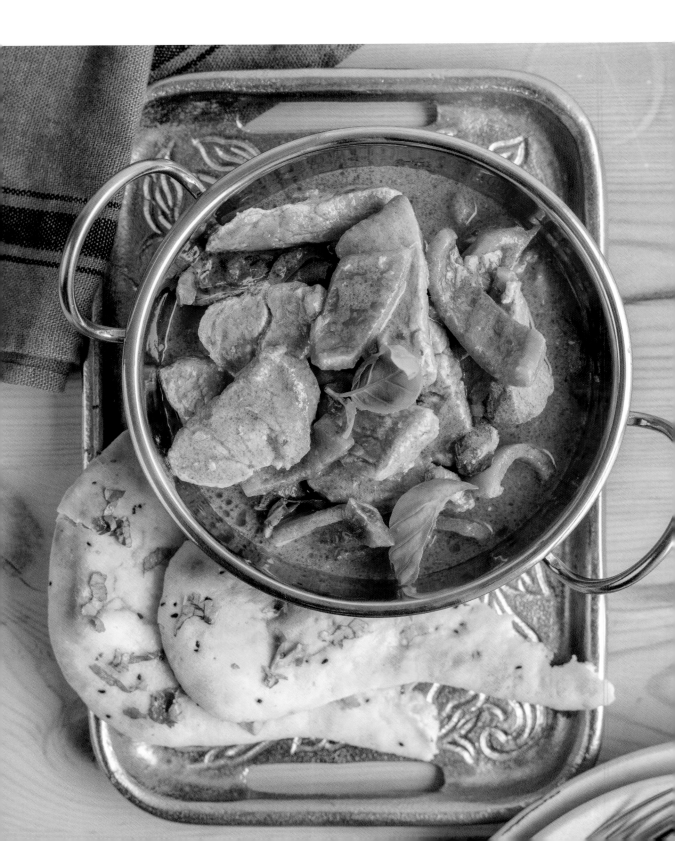

RED PORK CURRY

423 CALORIES per serving

Pork is much cheaper than chicken and beef and just as versatile. I often cook a pork fillet as it's very lean and tasty too. This is a cracking curry that tastes extremely fresh and fragrant and is a great choice midweek as it doesn't take long to prepare or cook. Serve with rice or extra vegetables.

INGREDIENTS

500g pork fillet, sliced
Pinch of black pepper
1 tsp coconut oil
3 spring onions, chopped
1 green pepper, sliced
2 garlic cloves, finely chopped
2 tsp minced ginger
200g red Thai curry paste (may need more or less depending on how spicy your paste is and your taste)
400ml light coconut milk
1 tbsp fish sauce
1 tbsp dark soy sauce
1 tsp sugar
Handful of fresh basil leaves

Season the pork fillet with black pepper, then heat the coconut oil in a wok on a high heat.

Add the pork, spring onion and green pepper and fry for a few minutes. Add the garlic and ginger and fry for a further minute.

Add the curry paste and fry for about 30 seconds before pouring in the coconut milk, fish sauce, soy sauce and sugar.

Reduce the heat and simmer for around 5 minutes or until the curry starts to thicken. Stir through the basil leaves then serve.

Prep time: 10 minutes
Cook time: 10 minutes
Serves: 3

7 925414 000770

Nutritional info per serving:
Calories: 423kcal
Protein 40g
Carbs 14g
Fat 23g

PORK *in a* PINT CASSEROLE

517
CALORIES
per serving

This is a delicious, easy-to-make pork and cider casserole that's creamy, popular with the kids (at least in our household) but is equally good as a dinner party crowd-pleaser.

INGREDIENTS

1 tbsp olive oil
200g unsmoked bacon (fat removed), chopped
2 red onions, sliced
2 carrots, chopped
3 garlic cloves, crushed
1kg pork fillet, chopped
30g cornflour
1 tbsp mixed herbs
2 tsp wholegrain mustard
500ml medium or dry cider
250ml chicken stock
2 apples (not cooking variety), cored and sliced
100ml reduced-fat crème fraîche

Preheat the oven to 160°C (140°C fan)/315°F/gas 3.

Heat the olive oil in a large ovenproof dish and fry the bacon, onion and carrot for around 5 minutes or until cooked. Add the garlic and fry for 30 seconds more.

Add the pork and the cornflour and mix through. Add the mixed herbs, mustard, cider, stock and apple to the dish and combine.

Bake in the oven for around 3 hours. Remove from the oven, stir through the crème fraîche and serve.

Nutritional info per serving:
Calories: 517kcal
Protein: 61g
Carbs: 21g
Fat: 21g

Prep time: 20 minutes
Cook time: 3 hours 15 minutes
Serves: 5

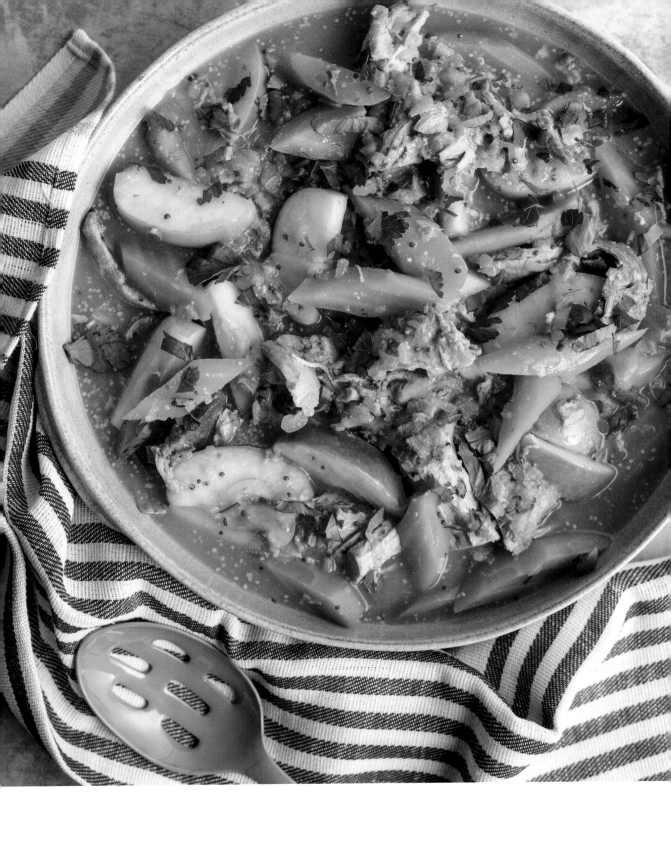

PORK SCHNITZEL
with POTATO SALAD

517
CALORIES
per serving

I do love a good schnitzel. Crunchy, meaty, yummy. Nuff said. These are cooked in the air fryer but if you don't have one, they can be pan-fried or cooked in the oven. If you don't like pork then chicken is a perfect substitute in this recipe. Prepare and cook it exactly the same way. The potato salad works well with schnitzels and is a popular accompaniment to them in Germany and Austria. It also goes well with other recipes that you might eat in summer or cook on a barbecue, such as the Best DIY Burger.

INGREDIENTS

4 pork loin steaks (about 125g each)
15g plain flour
70g panko breadcrumbs
1 egg, beaten

Potato salad

600g baby new potatoes (unpeeled)
1 tsp olive oil
3 bacon medallions, chopped
1 red onion, sliced
1 tsp minced garlic
1 tsp apple cider vinegar
15g Dijon mustard
15g mayonnaise
35g Greek yoghurt
Small handful of fresh parsley
Few grinds of black pepper

Boil the potatoes for 15–20 minutes until cooked through, then drain.

For the pork, bash each of the steaks with a rolling pin until they are thin – about 1cm. Place the flour on one plate, the breadcrumbs on another and the egg in a bowl. Dip the steaks into the flour first, then the egg, then the breadcrumbs and set aside.

Cook the pork for 12 minutes at 200°C in the air fryer. If you don't have one, you can pan-fry with a little olive oil, oven bake or grill.

For the potato salad, heat the olive oil in a frying pan on a medium heat and fry the bacon, onion and garlic until the bacon starts to brown. Remove from the heat and put in a bowl along with the apple cider vinegar, Dijon mustard, mayonnaise, Greek yoghurt, parsley and black pepper.

Add the cooked potatoes to the bowl and mix through so they're coated in the mixture. Serve.

**Nutritional info
per serving:**
Calories: 517kcal
Protein: 51g
Carbs: 40g
Fat: 17g

Prep time: 20 minutes
Cook time: 20 minutes
Serves: 4

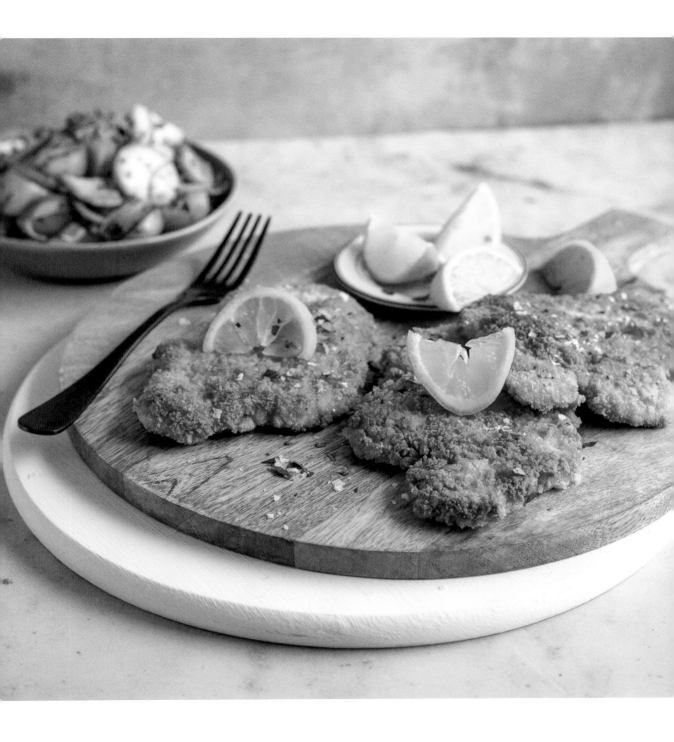

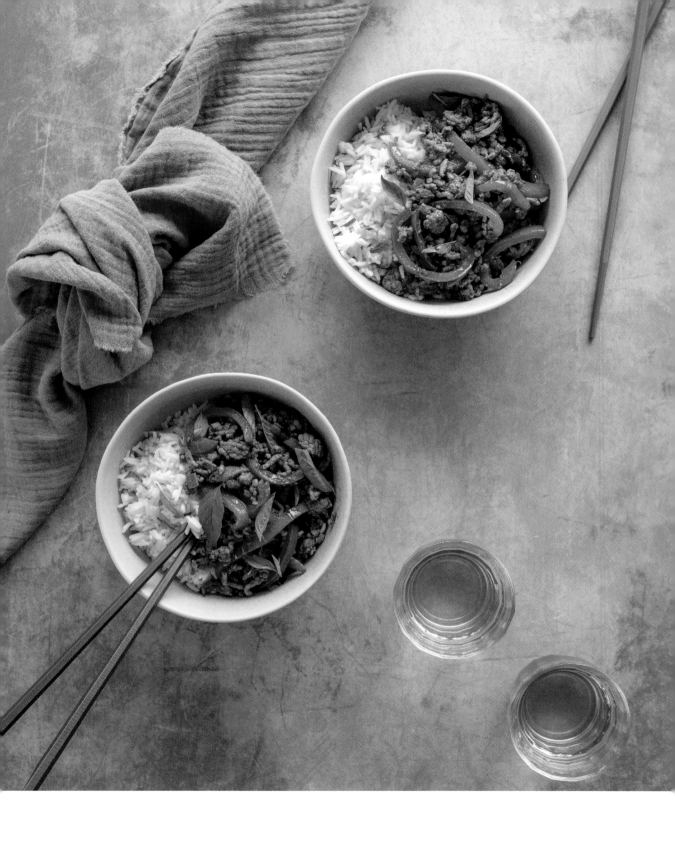

THAI BASIL PORK
(PAD KRA PAO)

Pad Kra Pao or Thai Basil Pork is an extremely popular recipe served and enjoyed all over Thailand. This is what happens when you go out for Thai food, discover a new recipe, love it, then want to be able to make restaurant-quality food in your own home. There are several things that make this Pad Kra Pao recipe so appealing: it's extremely tasty, it takes less than 15 minutes to cook and it's roughly 200 calories per serving. What a combo.

INGREDIENTS

2 tbsp coconut oil
1 red pepper, finely chopped
4 spring onions, finely chopped
1 green chilli, finely chopped
5g garlic, mashed
5g ginger, mashed
500g 5%-fat pork mince
1 tbsp fish sauce
1 tbsp soy sauce
100ml water
1 tsp honey
Handful of fresh Thai basil leaves

Over a high heat, add 1 tsp of coconut oil to a wok and add the pork mince. Cook for 8-10 minutes until it really starts to brown and take on a delicious flavour.

Remove the pork from the wok once cooked, return the wok to the stove and reduce to a medium heat. Add the remaining 1 tsp coconut oil along with the red pepper and spring onions. Fry for a minute or so until they start to soften.

Add the chilli, ginger and garlic and fry for a further 30 seconds.

Add the fish sauce, soy sauce, water and honey, and simmer for a couple of minutes.

Mix through the basil until it wilts then serve.

Prep time: 10 minutes
Cook time: 15 minutes
Serves: 4

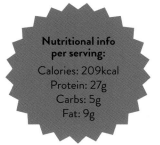

Nutritional info
per serving:
Calories: 209kcal
Protein: 27g
Carbs: 5g
Fat: 9g

SPICY KOREAN BULGOGI PORK

Bulgogi is a winner of a stir-fry recipe for midweek and it works just as well with thin steak slices if you're looking for an alternative to pork. Traditionally you'd use gochujang paste (Korean chilli paste). If you've got some, great – if not, no problem at all, just follow my ingredients list below. For side dishes, the obvious companion to this one is rice and any kind of vegetable. This recipe is best eaten fresh as you'll find the sauce disappears if you try and reheat it from frozen.

INGREDIENTS

Marinade

2 tsp minced ginger
2 garlic cloves, crushed
60ml reduced-salt soy sauce
1 tbsp rice wine vinegar or white wine vinegar
1 tbsp sesame oil
1 tsp chilli flakes
15g honey

500g pork fillet, cut into thin strips
1 tsp sesame oil
1 green pepper, thinly sliced
1 carrot, thinly sliced
4 spring onions, thinly sliced

Mix all the marinade ingredients together and marinate the pork for at least an hour.

Heat the sesame oil in a frying pan.

Drain the pork, reserving the marinade.

Add the veg and meat to the pan and cook over a high heat until cooked through. Add the marinade and heat through. Serve with rice, or stir-fried tenderstem broccoli and mangetouts.

Nutritional info per serving:

Calories: 349kcal
Protein: 38g
Carbs: 11g
Fat: 17g

Prep time: 10 minutes + 1 hour to marinate
Cook time: 10 minutes
Serves: 3

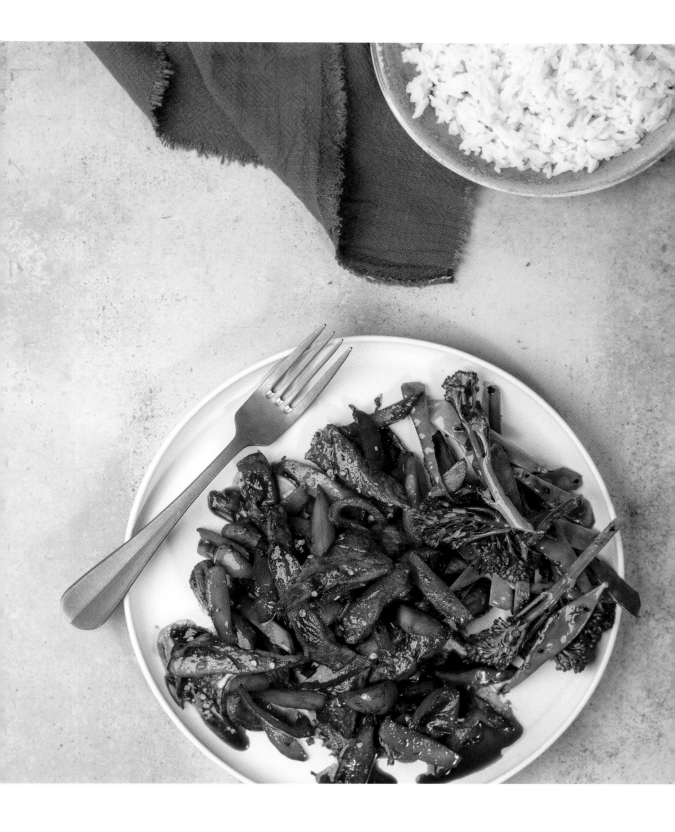

SPANISH MEATBALLS

There's a mistaken idea that meatballs take too long to make and that you can achieve the same taste by just making a Bolognese. That couldn't be further from the truth. Meatballs offer a really satisfying mouthful, a delish vehicle for all sorts of sauces, and you get the added satisfaction of seeing them hold together in the cooking. Follow this method and they should do that nicely.

INGREDIENTS

2 tbsp olive oil
½ onion, very finely chopped
2 garlic cloves, chopped
20g small capers, chopped
1 tbsp paprika
1 tbsp dried oregano
500g 5%-fat pork mince
50g reduced-fat chorizo, very finely chopped
80g breadcrumbs
50g low-fat mild cheddar cheese, grated
1 egg
15g fresh parsley, chopped (add more for garnish)
500g tomato-based pasta sauce from a jar (or make your own)
Salt and pepper

Heat a non-stick frying pan to medium and pour in 1 tablespoon of olive oil. Add the onion, garlic and capers and cook for 10 minutes, until the onion is translucent.

In a bowl, combine the paprika, oregano, pork mince, chorizo, breadcrumbs, cheese, egg, parsley, salt and pepper and the cooked onion/garlic/caper mixture. Mix until all ingredients are combined. Spoon out the meat and use your hands to form it into meatballs, about the size of a golf ball.

Heat a non-stick frying pan to medium and add the rest of the olive oil. Cook the meatballs until golden brown on every side. Once they are golden, add the tomato sauce, heat through and serve.

Nutritional info per serving:
Calories: 442kcal
Protein: 37g
Carbs: 24g
Fat: 22g

Prep time: 15 minutes
Cook time: 30 minutes
Serves: 4

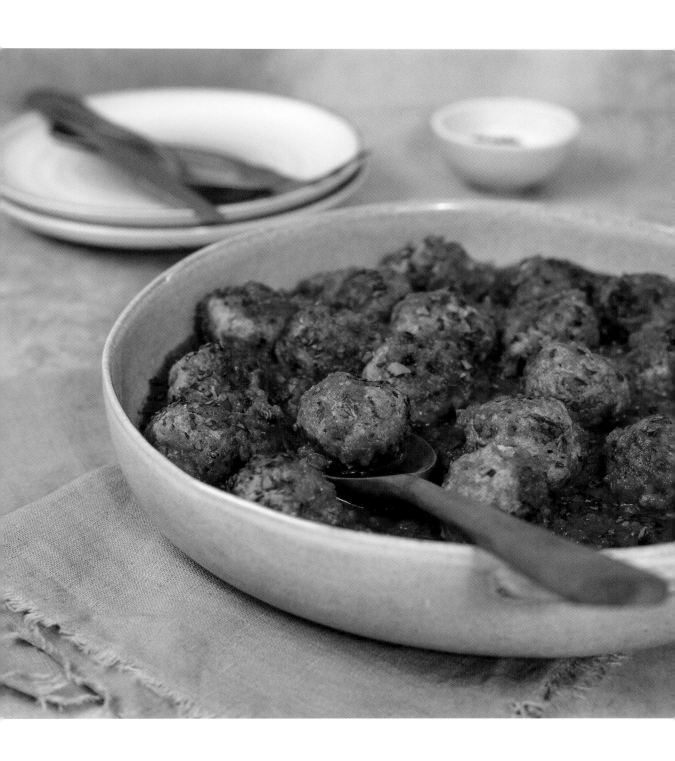

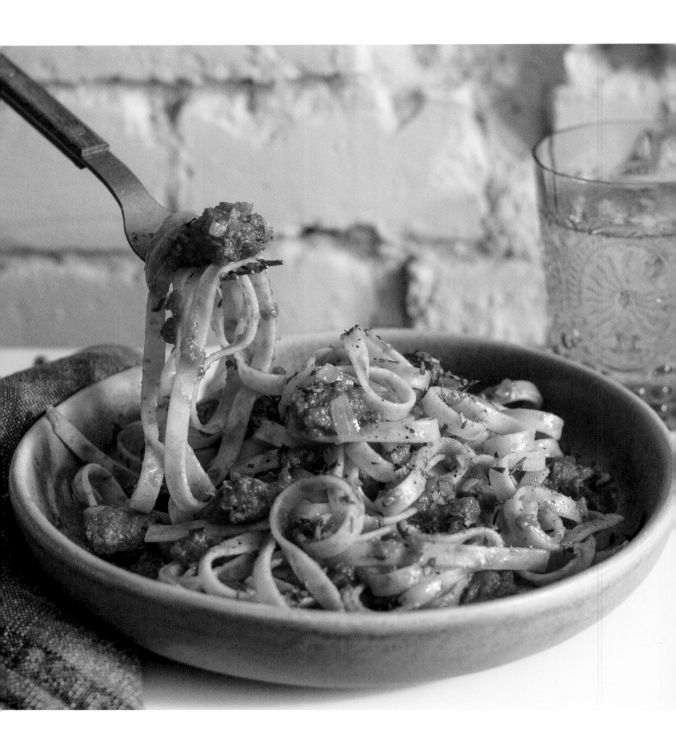

SPICY VENISON SAUSAGE RAGU

A rich, warming recipe that's great for autumn and winter nights when you need some comfort food. It goes really well with pasta and a glass of red, if you so choose. If you can't get your hands on venison sausages, just go for lean beef sausages instead.

INGREDIENTS

1 tsp olive oil
1 onion, chopped
500g venison sausages, chopped
1 garlic clove, crushed
300g hot salsa
2 tbsp tomato pesto
400g tin chopped tomatoes
½ tsp dried rosemary
Salt and pepper

Heat the olive oil in a large pan over a medium heat and fry the onion and sausages until cooked through and turning golden brown. Add the garlic and fry for a minute more.

Add all the remaining ingredients, reduce the heat to low and simmer for 15 minutes.

Serve with your choice of pasta.

Prep time: 10 minutes
Cook time: 30 minutes
Serves: 4

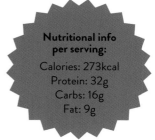

Nutritional info
per serving:
Calories: 273kcal
Protein: 32g
Carbs: 16g
Fat: 9g

MEDITERRANEAN BAKED FISH

479 CALORIES per serving

This will bring back lovely summer holiday memories of sun-drenched lunches and sunset dinners beside the sea. It's colourful, healthy, delicious and one of the best ways to get a big protein hit.

INGREDIENTS

1kg skinned firm white fish fillets, eg haddock or cod, cut into large chunks
Juice of 1 lemon
1 tbsp olive oil
3 onions, thinly sliced
4 garlic cloves, crushed
900g ripe tomatoes, chopped
2 tbsp tomato purée
Pinch of sugar
Pinch of chilli flakes
1 tsp dried oregano
120ml red wine
12 black pitted olives
Handful of fresh flat-leaf parsley, chopped
800g boiled potatoes
Salt and pepper

Put the fish in a large ovenproof baking dish. Drizzle with the lemon juice and season with salt and pepper. Cover and set aside to marinate in a cool place for 30 minutes.

Preheat the oven to 180°C (160°C fan)/350°F/gas 4.

Heat the oil in a large frying pan set over a low to medium heat. Cook the onion and garlic, stirring occasionally, for 8–10 minutes, or until tender. Add the tomatoes, tomato purée, sugar, chilli flakes, oregano and wine. Cook, uncovered, for 10–15 minutes until the sauce thickens and reduces. Stir in the olives and most of the parsley.

Pour the sauce over the fish and bake in the preheated oven for 20–25 minutes, or until the fish is cooked and opaque. Sprinkle with the remaining parsley and serve immediately with boiled potatoes.

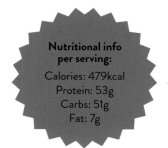

Nutritional info per serving:
Calories: 479kcal
Protein: 53g
Carbs: 51g
Fat: 7g

Prep time: 10 minutes + 30 minutes to marinate
Cook time: 40–50 minutes
Serves: 4

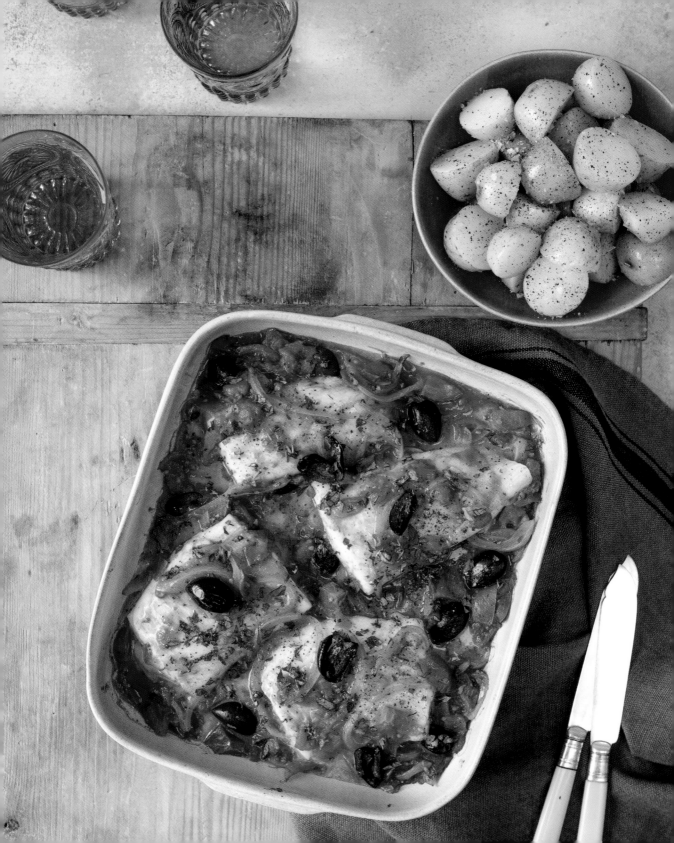

BLACK COD *with* SESAME NOODLES

496 CALORIES per serving

There's no need to eat out in a smart restaurant when you can enjoy this Japanese fakeaway at home. It's easy to make and great for entertaining. Just prepare the cod a day in advance so it absorbs the distinctive flavours of the miso marinade before cooking.

INGREDIENTS

4 x 200g thick cod (or other white fish) fillets, skinned
Olive oil, for brushing
250g frozen edamame beans
½ tsp chilli flakes
½ tsp sea salt flakes
½ tsp sesame oil, plus extra for drizzling
300g rice noodles (dry weight)
4 tsp pickled ginger
4 spring onions, shredded
Sesame seeds, for sprinkling

Marinade

4 tbsp sake (Japanese rice wine)
4 tbsp mirin
6 tsp caster sugar
4 tbsp white miso paste

Make the marinade: heat the sake, mirin and sugar in a small pan set over a high heat. Stir gently to dissolve the sugar and when it starts to boil, turn the heat down to low and stir in the miso. Keep stirring until it dissolves and then take the pan off the heat.

When the marinade is cool, pour it into a container large enough to hold the fish and add the cod fillets, turning them until they are lightly coated with the marinade. Cover with a lid or cling film and marinate in the fridge overnight.

The following day, pat the cod dry with kitchen paper. Lightly brush a large frying pan with oil and set over a medium to high heat. When the pan is hot, add the cod and cook for 2–3 minutes, or until brown underneath. Turn the fillets over carefully and cook for 2–3 minutes on the other side.

Place the pan under a preheated hot overhead grill or in a preheated oven at 200°C (180°C fan)/400°F/gas 6 and cook for 5–10 minutes, or until the cod is flaky and cooked right through.

Meanwhile, cook the frozen edamame beans in a pan of boiling water as directed on the packet, then drain. Mix the hot beans with the chilli flakes, salt and sesame oil.

Cook the rice noodles as directed on the packet.

Serve the black cod garnished with the pickled ginger and spring onions, with the edamame beans and rice noodles, drizzled with sesame oil (if wished) and sprinkled with sesame seeds.

Nutritional info per serving:
Calories: 496kcal
Protein: 43g
Carbs: 54g
Fat: 12g

Prep time: 15 minutes + overnight to marinate
Cook time: 15 minutes
Serves: 4

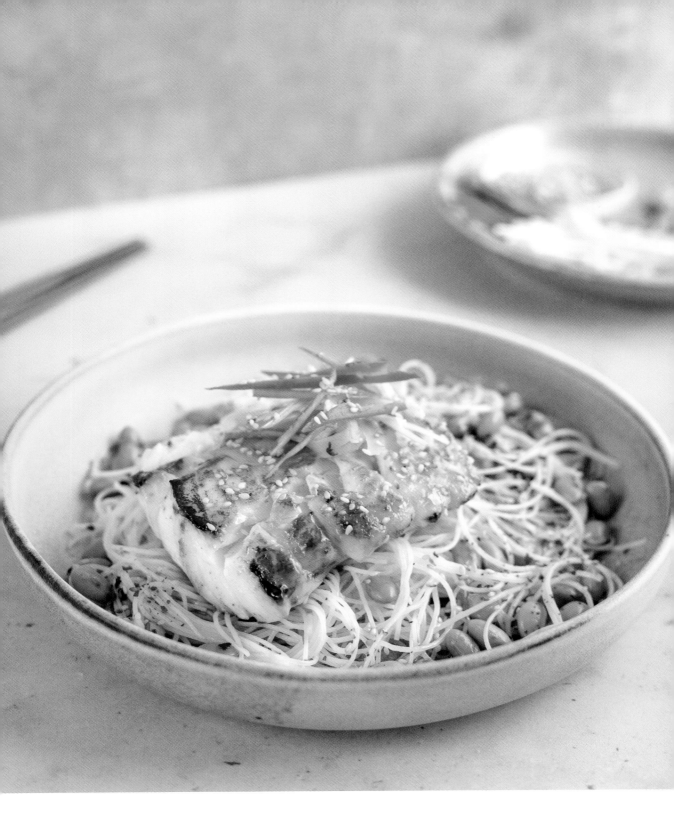

QUICK *and* EASY CHEESY VEGETABLE PIE

497 CALORIES per serving

This vegetable pie is tasty, economical and easy to make. It's also perfect for a cold winter's evening and a great way to use up vegetables lurking at the back of the fridge. Any combination of root vegetables is suitable for the vegetable mash – whatever you have handy.

INGREDIENTS

2 tbsp olive oil
1 onion, finely chopped
2 garlic cloves, crushed
2 leeks, washed, trimmed and thickly sliced
400g mushrooms, quartered
400g tin cannellini or butter beans, rinsed and drained
200g spinach leaves, washed, trimmed and shredded
4 tbsp grated low-fat cheddar cheese

Vegetable mash

1kg mixed potatoes, sweet potatoes, parsnips, swede, peeled and cubed
30g butter
60ml milk
150g grated low-fat cheddar cheese
Salt and pepper

Preheat the oven to 200°C (180°C fan)/400°F/gas 6.

Make the vegetable mash: put the cubed vegetables in a large pan of salted water and bring to the boil. Reduce the heat and simmer gently for 10–15 minutes until cooked and tender. Drain well and return the vegetables to the hot pan. Mash with the butter and milk until there are no lumps. Add some black pepper and stir in the grated cheese.

Meanwhile, heat the oil in a large frying pan set over a low to medium heat and cook the onion, garlic and leeks, stirring occasionally, for 8–10 minutes until softened. Add the mushrooms and cook for 3–4 minutes until golden. Add the beans and cook for 2–3 minutes more. Stir in the spinach and cook for 1 minute until it wilts.

Cover the base of a shallow ovenproof dish with half the vegetable mash, then spoon the cooked leek and mushroom filling over the top. Cover with the remaining mashed vegetables and rough up the top with a fork. Sprinkle with grated cheddar.

Bake in the preheated oven for 20–25 minutes, or until golden brown and crisp on top. Serve immediately.

Nutritional info per serving:
Calories: 497kcal
Protein: 26g
Carbs: 51g
Fat: 21g

Prep time: 20 minutes
Cook time: 40–45 minutes
Serves: 5

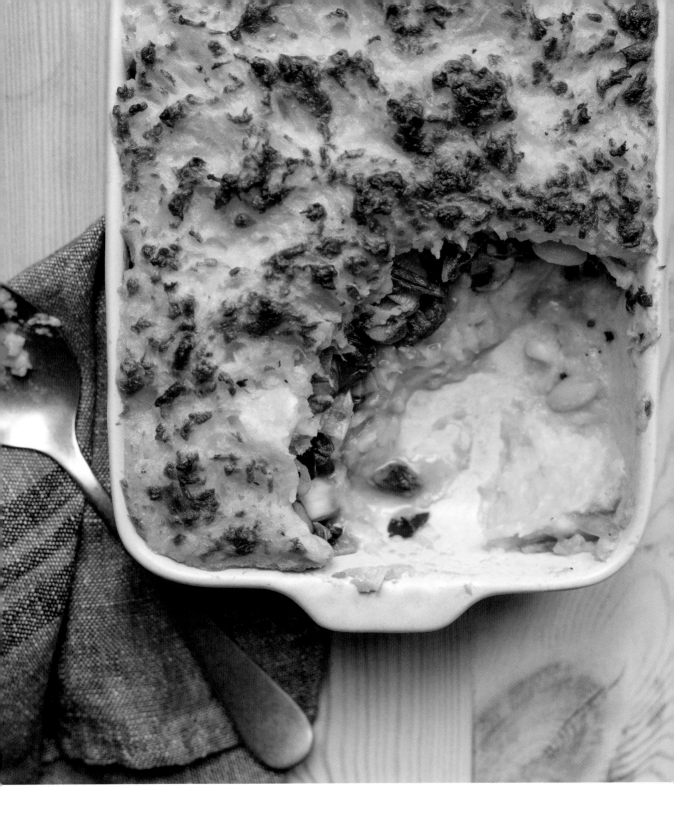

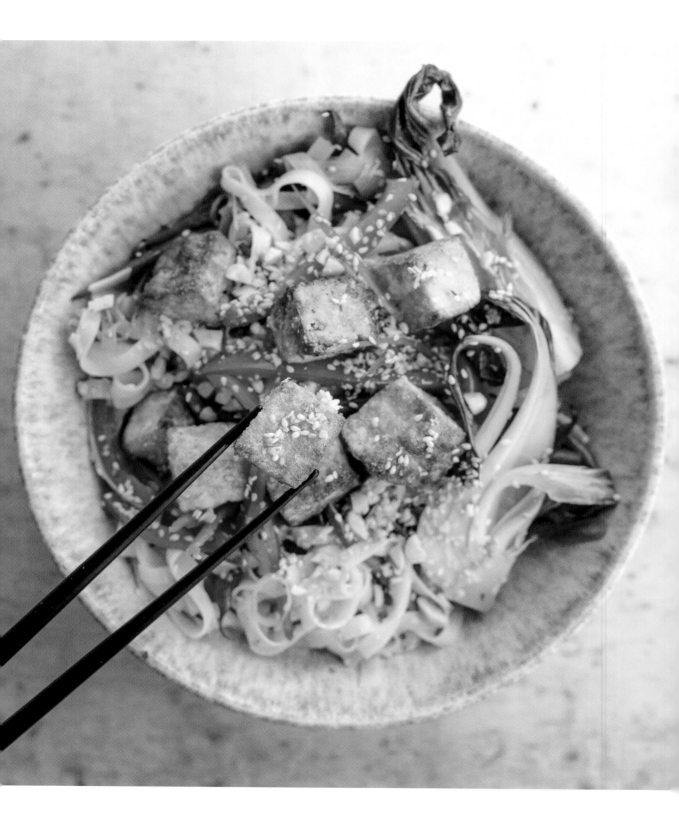

STIR-FRIED CRISPY TOFU

This vegan stir-fry is great for a quick supper when you get home from work. Tofu (soya bean curd) is a healthy source of plant protein. It's low in fat and carbs but packed with essential minerals, especially iron and calcium.

INGREDIENTS

600g firm tofu, drained and cubed (always use firm tofu for stir-fries as it keeps its shape)

3 tbsp cornflour

2 tbsp coconut oil

2.5cm piece of ginger, peeled and grated

3 garlic cloves, thinly sliced

1 hot red chilli, shredded

Bunch of spring onions, thinly sliced

2 red peppers, thinly sliced

150g fine green beans, trimmed

2 pak choi, cut into quarters lengthways

500g fresh ready-to-cook rice noodles

4 tbsp dark soy sauce

Juice of 1 lime

4 tbsp roasted salted peanuts, chopped

Sesame seeds, for sprinkling

Salt and pepper

Pat the tofu dry with kitchen paper and lightly dust with cornflour seasoned with salt and pepper. Heat the oil in a wok or a deep frying pan set over a medium to high heat and stir-fry the tofu in batches for 4–5 minutes until crispy and golden. Remove and drain on kitchen paper. Keep warm.

Reduce the heat to medium and stir-fry the ginger, garlic, chilli and spring onion for 1 minute. Add the peppers and green beans and stir-fry for 2–3 minutes.

Add the pak choi and noodles and stir-fry for 2–3 minutes or until the noodles are heated through and the pak choi is just tender but still a little crisp. Toss with the soy sauce and lime juice.

Divide between four shallow bowls and top with the crispy tofu and peanuts. Sprinkle with sesame seeds and serve piping hot.

Prep time: 15 minutes
Cook time: 10–12 minutes
Serves: 4

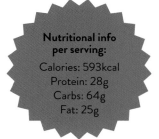

Nutritional info
per serving:
Calories: 593kcal
Protein: 28g
Carbs: 64g
Fat: 25g

PART 4
HEALTHY

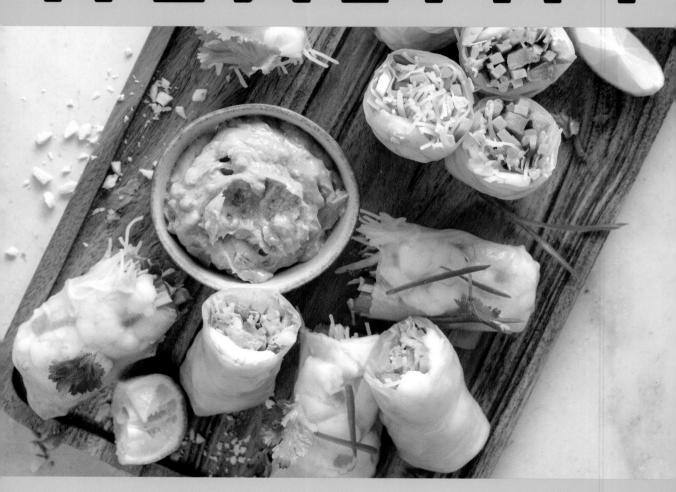

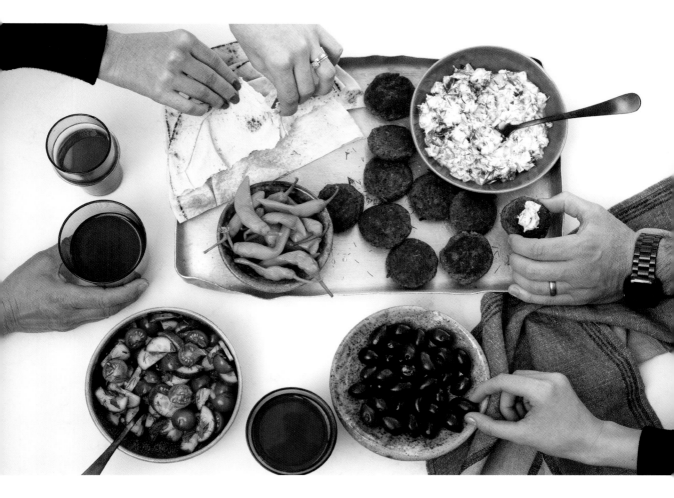

SNACKS

THE *Ultimate* HIGH PROTEIN HANDBOOK

WHEN YOU'RE LOOKING FOR A WEE PROTEIN SOMETHING TO NIBBLE ON, YOU CAN GIVE THESE RECIPES A TRY. THERE'S SWEET SNACKS LIKE YUMMY RASPBERRY YOGHURT MUFFINS THROUGH TO SAVOURY OPTIONS LIKE CARROT FALAFELS WITH A DELICIOUS TZATZIKI DIP THAT WOULD ALSO BE A LOVELY ADDITION TO THE ZA'ATAR CHICKEN.

CRUNCHY PEANUT BUTTER SQUARES

431
CALORIES
per square

Nibble these crunchy peanut butter squares as a delicious power snack when you need to boost your protein or you're experiencing mid-morning hunger pangs. You can vary the seeds: try linseed, flax and poppy seeds. You could also use dried cranberries or chopped dates instead of raisins.

INGREDIENTS

115g butter
115g crunchy peanut butter
4 tbsp clear honey
2 large, overripe bananas, mashed
350g porridge oats
100g ready-to-eat dried apricots, chopped
30g raisins
60g mixed seeds, eg chia, sunflower,
  pumpkin, sesame seeds
Pinch of sea salt crystals

Preheat the oven to 160°C (140°C fan)/315°F/gas 3. Lightly butter a 20cm square shallow baking tin and line with greaseproof paper.

Put the butter, peanut butter and honey in a pan set over a low heat and stir until everything has melted and combined.

Remove from the heat and stir in the bananas, oats, dried fruit, seeds and a pinch of salt. If the mixture is not firm enough, add some more oats; if it's not sticky enough, add more honey.

Spoon into the prepared tin, pressing down well on the mixture with the back of a metal spoon to level the top. Bake for 25 minutes or until crisp and golden brown.

Leave to cool in the tin before cutting into squares. Transfer to an airtight container and store in a cool place for up to 4 days.

**Nutritional info
per square:**
Calories: 431kcal
Protein: 10g
Carbs: 46g
Fat: 23g

Prep time: 10 minutes
Cook time: 25 minutes
Makes: 9 squares

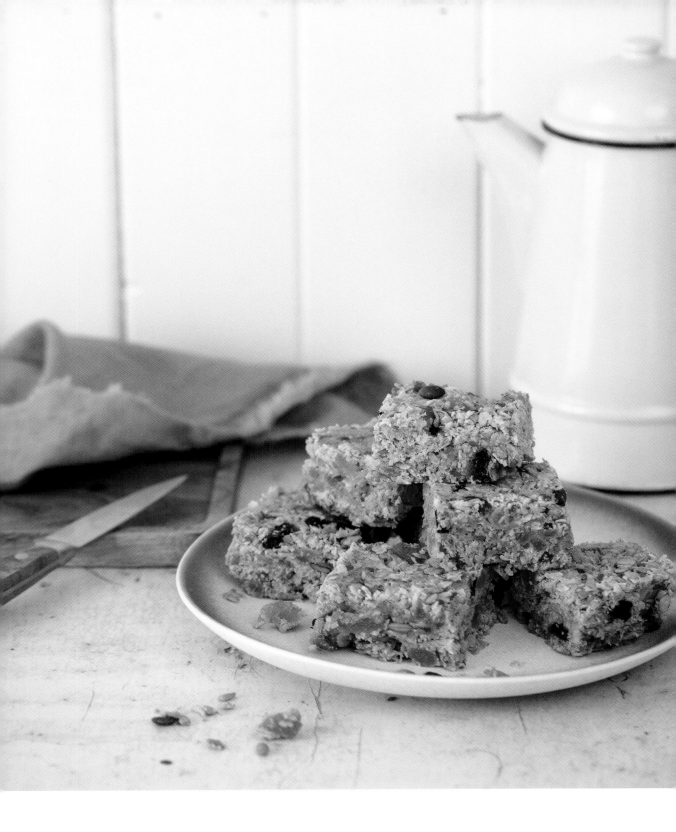

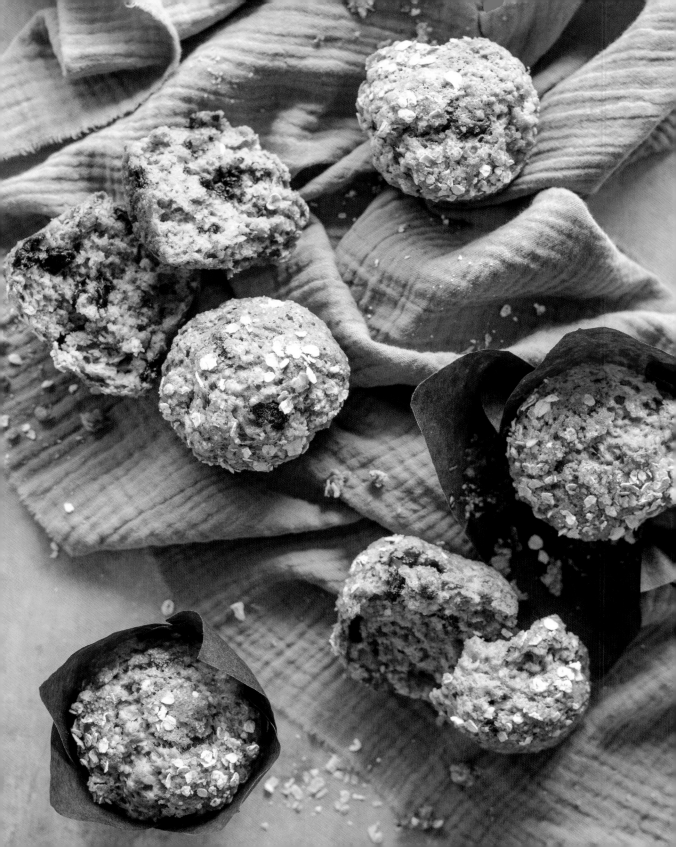

NUTTY BANANA OAT MUFFINS

These crunchy muffins, studded with chocolate chips and nuts, are healthy and delicious. Plus, they're so easy to make – you don't need any special equipment. They are irresistible and just two muffins will supply 14 grams of protein. To test whether the muffins are cooked, insert a thin metal skewer into the middle of one. It should come out clean. A wee smidge of orange zest is also a great addition.

INGREDIENTS

115g porridge oats, plus extra for sprinkling
200g wholewheat flour
1½ tsp baking powder
1 tsp bicarbonate of soda
½ tsp sea salt
1 tsp ground cinnamon
115g light brown sugar
4 medium bananas
2 medium free-range eggs, beaten
60ml olive oil
4 tbsp milk
Few drops of vanilla extract
115g chopped walnuts
4 tbsp dark chocolate chips
4 tbsp sesame seeds
1 tsp demerera sugar

Preheat the oven to 180°C (160°C fan)/350°F/gas 4. Line a 12-hole muffin pan with paper cases.

Mix the oats, flour, baking powder, bicarbonate of soda, salt, cinnamon and sugar in a large bowl and make a hollow in the centre. Mash the bananas with a fork and mix with the beaten eggs, oil, milk and vanilla in a smaller bowl.

Pour the banana mixture into the hollow in the oat mixture and stir gently. Fold in the nuts, chocolate chips and seeds, being careful not to overmix. Divide between the paper cases and sprinkle a little demerera sugar and a few oats over the top.

Bake the muffins for 20 minutes, or until slightly risen and golden brown. Leave to cool and eat slightly warm or store in an airtight container in the fridge for 2–3 days. They freeze well for up to 3 months.

Prep time: 15 minutes
Cook time: 20 minutes
Makes: 12 muffins

Nutritional info per muffin:
Calories: 338kcal
Protein: 7g
Carbs: 37g
Fat: 18g

RASPBERRY YOGHURT MUFFINS

218
CALORIES
per muffin

I like to use raspberries instead of the more familiar blueberries in muffins to mix things up a bit, partly because I always get plenty from my garden. As a note, the longer you beat the butter and sugar, the lighter the muffins will be. Don't worry if the mixture curdles when you add the eggs. It won't make any difference to the results. Also, adding some protein powder to the mix boosts the content even more.

INGREDIENTS

100g butter, softened
150g caster sugar
2 large free-range eggs
150g 0%-fat Greek yoghurt
3 tbsp milk
Few drops of vanilla extract
75g vanilla whey protein powder
175g plain flour
2 tsp baking powder
1 tsp bicarbonate of soda
2 tbsp chia seeds
3 tbsp poppy seeds
¼ tsp salt
100g fresh raspberries

Preheat the oven to 180°C (160°C fan)/350°F/gas 4. Line a 12-hole muffin pan with paper cases.

Beat the butter and sugar in a food mixer, or with an electric hand-held whisk, until light and fluffy. Beat in the eggs, one at a time, and then add the yoghurt, milk and vanilla extract.

Put the protein powder in a bowl and sift in the flour, baking powder and bicarbonate of soda. Stir in the seeds and salt. Add to the yoghurt mixture and fold in gently with a metal spoon in a figure-of-eight motion. The mixture should be neither too stiff nor too liquid. If it's too stiff, add more milk; too liquid, add more flour. Gently fold in the raspberries, distributing them evenly throughout the mixture.

Spoon into the paper cases and bake for 20 minutes, or until the muffins are well-risen and golden brown. Insert a fine metal skewer into a muffin to test whether it is cooked – it should come out clean. Leave in the muffin pan for a few minutes before cooling on a wire rack.

Store the muffins in a sealed airtight container. They will keep well for 3 days. They can also be frozen for up to 1 month.

Nutritional info per muffin:
Calories: 218kcal
Protein: 7g
Carbs: 25g
Fat: 10g

Prep time: 15 minutes
Cook time: 20 minutes
Makes: 12 muffins

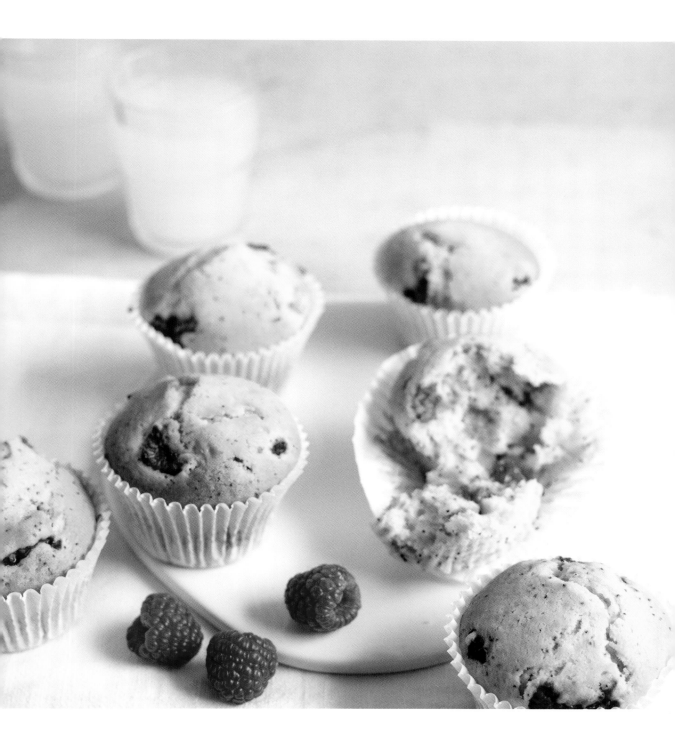

SEEDY PROTEIN BALLS

98
CALORIES
per ball

These bite-sized balls are perfect for when you need a quick power snack or energy boost. Just grab a couple and eat them on the go. They are very versatile and you can swap some of the ingredients for your favourite nut butter, sweetener, seeds or dried fruit.

INGREDIENTS

175g peanut butter (crunchy or smooth)
6 tbsp maple syrup or agave
1 tsp vanilla extract
175g porridge oats
30g chia seeds
30g dried blueberries or cranberries
60g dark chocolate chips (minimum 70% cocoa solids)
4 tbsp sesame seeds

Line a large baking tray with greaseproof paper.

Put the peanut butter and maple syrup or agave into a medium-sized saucepan set over a low heat and stir. When they combine, take the pan off the heat.

Stir in the vanilla extract and then mix in the oats, chia seeds, dried fruit and chocolate chips. If the mixture is too sticky and wet, add some more oats; if it's too dry, add a little cold water.

Take small spoonfuls of the mixture and, using your hands, roll them into small bite-sized balls. Put the sesame seeds in a shallow container and roll the balls around in the seeds until they are coated.

Place the balls on the lined baking tray and chill in the fridge for 2 hours or until set. Store them in an airtight container in the fridge. They will keep well for 1 week.

Nutritional info per ball:
Calories: 98kcal
Protein: 3g
Carbs: 8g
Fat: 6g

Prep time: 15 minutes
Chill: 2 hours
Makes: 30 balls

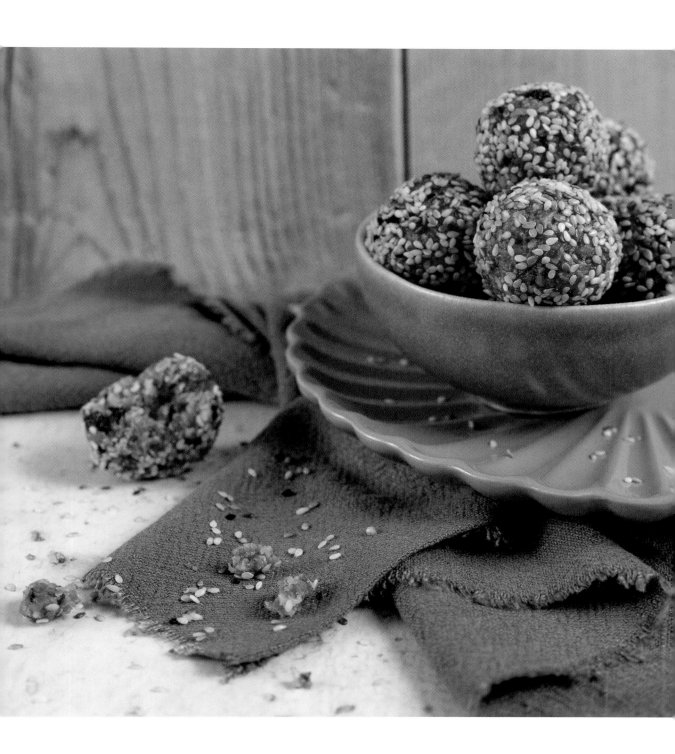

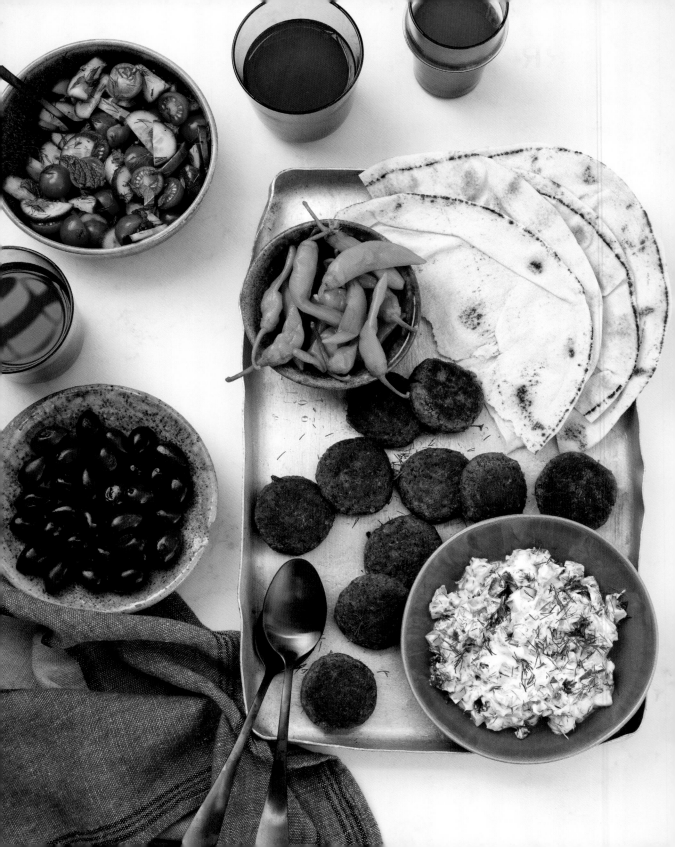

CARROT FALAFELS
with TZATZIKI

70
CALORIES
per falafel

Falafels are a tasty way to snack on some vegetable protein (chickpeas). Keep some in a sealed container in the fridge for when you're feeling peckish, or make double the quantity and enjoy them served with salad in a pita bread or wrap for lunch.

INGREDIENTS

60g carrot, finely grated
400g tin chickpeas, drained and rinsed
3 spring onions, thinly sliced
1 green chilli, diced
1 garlic clove, crushed
Grated zest of 1 lemon
Handful of fresh coriander, finely chopped
30g plain flour
½ tsp baking powder
1 tsp cumin seeds
1 tsp coriander seeds
Sunflower oil, for shallow frying
Sea salt and pepper

Tzatziki
250g 0%-fat Greek yoghurt
1 tbsp olive oil
½ cucumber, diced
2 garlic cloves, crushed
Few sprigs of fresh mint and dill, chopped
Grated zest and juice of ½ lemon
Pinch of coarse sea salt crystals

Make the tzatziki: mix all the ingredients together in a bowl, adding salt to taste. Cover and chill in the fridge while you make the falafels.

To make the falafels, squeeze any excess moisture out of the carrot and pat dry with kitchen paper. Blitz in a food processor with the chickpeas, spring onions, chilli, garlic, lemon zest, coriander, flour, baking powder and seasoning.

Dry-fry the cumin and coriander seeds in a small frying pan set over a medium heat for 1 minute or until they release their aroma. Watch carefully so they don't catch and burn. Transfer to a food processor and blitz until everything is well combined.

Divide the mixture into 10 equal-sized portions and, using your hands, roll each one into a small ball.

Heat the oil in a large frying pan set over a medium to high heat and fry the falafels for 4–5 minutes, turning them occasionally, until crisp and golden brown. Remove and drain on kitchen paper. Serve hot or cold with the tzatziki.

**Nutritional info
per falafel:**

Calories: 70kcal
Protein: 5g
Carbs: 8g
Fat: 2g

Prep time: 25 minutes
Cook time: 5 minutes
Makes: 10 falafel

8 941302 687907

QUICK HOMEMADE HUMMUS *with* OATCAKES

435 CALORIES per serving

Why bother buying hummus when you can make it yourself? It's so quick and easy. Spread it on oatcakes or on wholegrain toast, add it to sandwiches or serve it with salad bowls and grilled meat, chicken and vegetables. It's infinitely versatile. For a pretty green version, add a handful of coriander or basil.

INGREDIENTS

2 x 400g tins chickpeas
4 tbsp tahini
2 garlic cloves, crushed
½ tsp ground cumin
2 tbsp olive oil, plus extra for drizzling
Juice of 1 large lemon, plus extra for drizzling
Pinch of sea salt crystals
Ground paprika, for dusting
2 tbsp toasted sunflower and pumpkin seeds
8 oatcakes, to serve

Drain the chickpeas, reserving some of the liquid, and rinse under cold running water in a colander. Drain and pat dry with kitchen paper.

Put most of the chickpeas, reserving a few for the garnish, in a blender or food processor with the tahini, garlic, cumin, olive oil and lemon juice. Blitz to a coarse purée.

Gradually add some of the reserved chickpea liquid or some extra olive oil or lemon juice through the feed tube until you end up with the consistency you want. It should be quite soft (but not runny) and a little grainy – not too smooth. Season to taste with salt.

Transfer the hummus to a serving bowl and drizzle with olive oil and more lemon juice. Dust with paprika and sprinkle with toasted seeds and the reserved whole chickpeas. Serve with oatcakes.

Store the hummus in a sealed container in the fridge. It will keep well for up to 3 days. Serve with vegetable crudités as well, eg carrot, red pepper and celery sticks, cauliflower florets and baby tomatoes.

Nutritional info per serving:
Calories: 435kcal
Protein: 16g
Carbs: 32g
Fat: 27g

Prep time: 15 minutes
Serves: 4

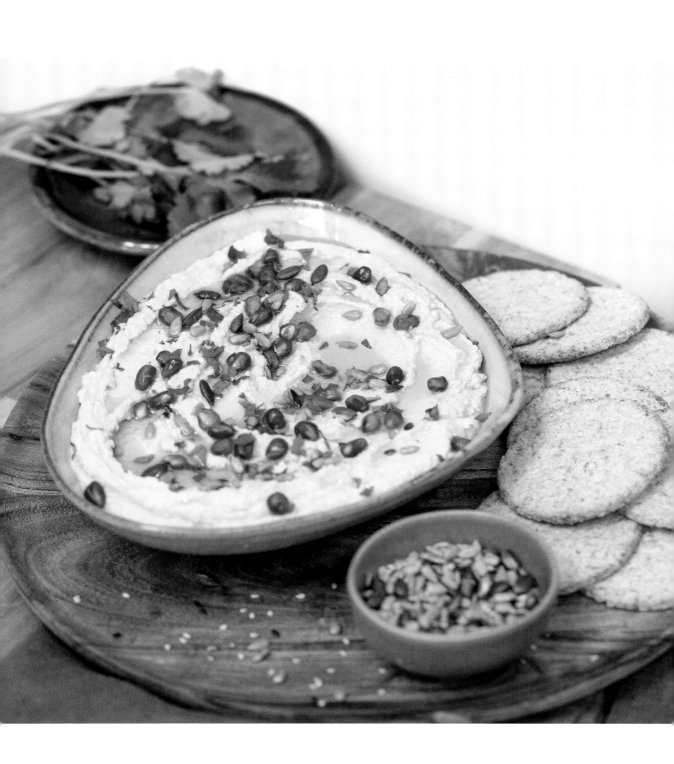

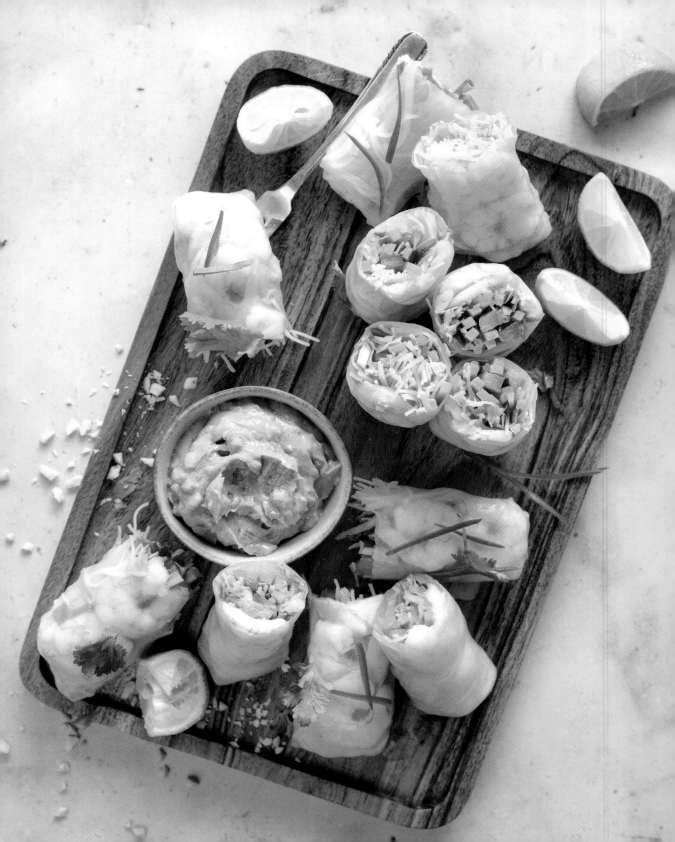

VIETNAMESE SPRING ROLLS

These delicious spring rolls are lighter and healthier than the more familiar fried ones. They are slightly fiddly to make but well worth the effort. Keep them fresh in the fridge in a sealed container for up to two days. You can buy rice paper wrappers in many Asian food shops, supermarkets and online. If you're not a fan of prawns, you can easily use chicken instead.

INGREDIENTS

60g rice vermicelli noodles (dry weight)
1 tsp sesame oil
1 tsp coconut oil
1 large red pepper, cut into thin strips
2 large carrots, cut into short thin
    matchsticks
100g shredded spring greens
100g bean sprouts
300g cooked peeled prawns
1 tsp minced ginger
2 tbsp light soy sauce
Handful of fresh coriander, chopped
Juice of 1 lime
1 avocado, peeled, stoned and diced
12 round rice paper wrappers

Peanut dipping sauce

100g crunchy peanut butter
2 garlic cloves, crushed
2 tbsp sweet chilli sauce
Juice of ½ lime
2 tbsp soy sauce
1 tbsp toasted sesame oil
1–2 tbsp water

Make the peanut dipping sauce: beat all the ingredients, except the water, in a bowl until they are well combined. Add the water, a tablespoon at a time, until you have a smooth and creamy sauce. Cover and chill until required.

Cook the rice noodles according to the instructions on the packet. Drain well and rinse under cold running water. Pat dry and toss in the sesame oil.

Heat the coconut oil in a wok or frying pan and stir-fry the red pepper and carrot for 2 minutes. Add the spring greens, bean sprouts and prawns and stir-fry for 2 minutes. Remove from the heat and stir in the ginger, soy sauce, coriander, lime juice and avocado. Once cooked, allow to cool for 10 minutes before handling.

Fill a bowl with cold water and dip a rice paper wrapper into it for 20 seconds, or until pliable. Lay it out flat and top with a few rice noodles and a spoonful of prawn and avocado filling, leaving a broad edge around the circle.

Fold the sides of the wrapper over the filling and roll up like a parcel. Repeat with the rest of the wrappers, rice noodles and filling until everything is used up. Serve with the peanut dipping sauce.

**Nutritional info
per spring roll:**
Calories: 188kcal
Protein: 11g
Carbs: 18g
Fat: 8g

Prep time: 30–40 minutes
Cook time: 10 minutes
Makes: 12 spring rolls

5 816997 064643

Recipe Notes

Recipe Notes

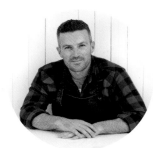

ACKNOWLEDGEMENTS

There's a lot of people I need to thank for making this book a reality.

First and foremost, thanks to my amazing followers and customers on Facebook, Instagram and my mailing list. If it weren't for you guys supporting me in my quest to get a 'real' book published, then it wouldn't have happened. Your reviews, comments, emails and general kind words all contributed to my publisher saying 'yes'.

Speaking of the publishers, thank you so much to the team at HarperNorth. In particular Jon, Gen, and Alice. I am so grateful you took a chance on me and made this book happen. Big thanks to my agent Sabhbh Curran at Curtis Brown for her continued support too.

In the kitchen, I'd like to thank Heather, Angela and Daisy for their help with the recipes, and thank you also to all my wonderful taste-testers who tried everything in this book. Special mention for Alison and her family, who provided extremely helpful feedback on so many of the meals.

Shout out to Georgie for her beautiful photos. They say the first bite is always with your eyes and I'd probably eat the entire book if that were the case. Thanks to Steph, my fantastic colleague for her continued excellent work and for making my job easier.

Lastly, and most importantly, thank you to my amazing family – Becky, Liliana and Maya – who are always at my side and make all of this worthwhile.

Follow me and find more recipes on my website
www.FoodForFitness.co.uk

WHEN USING KITCHEN APPLIANCES
PLEASE ALWAYS FOLLOW THE MANUFACTURER'S
INSTRUCTIONS

HarperNorth
Windmill Green
24 Mount Street
Manchester M2 3NX

HarperCollins*Publishers*
1 London Bridge Street
London SE1 9GF

www.harpercollins.co.uk

HarperCollins*Publishers*
Macken House, 39/40 Mayor Street Upper, Dublin 1
D01 C9W8 Ireland

First published by HarperCollins*Publishers* 2023

10 9 8 7 6 5 4 3 2 1

Text © Scott Baptie 2023
Photography © Georgie Glass 2023

Scott Baptie asserts the moral right to be identified as the author of this work

A catalogue record of this book is available from the British Library

ISBN 978-0-00-856305-9

Photography & Art Direction: Georgie Glass
Food Stylist: Angela Boggiano
Assistant Food Stylist: Daisy Hogg
Design and layout: Louise Leffler

Printed by GPS Group, Slovenia

All rights reserved. No part of this publication may be reproduced, stored in a retrieval system, or transmitted, in any form or by any means, electronic, mechanical, photocopying, recording or otherwise, without the prior written permission of the publishers.

The author of this work has made every effort to ensure that the information contained in this book is as accurate and up-to-date as possible at the time of publication. It is recommended that readers always consult a qualified medical specialist for individual advice, this book should not be used as an alternative to seeking specialist medical advice which should be sought before any action is taken. The author and publishers cannot be held responsible for any errors and omissions that may be found in the text, or any actions that may be taken by a reader as a result of any reliance on the information contained in the text which is taken entirely at the reader's own risk.

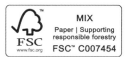

MIX
Paper | Supporting
responsible forestry
FSC™ C007454

This book is produced from independently certified FSC™ paper to ensure responsible forest management.

For more information visit: www.harpercollins.co.uk/green